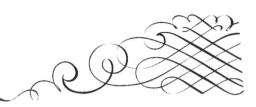
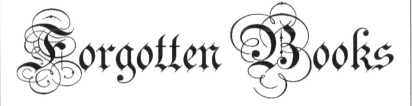
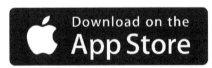
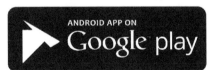

ISBN 978-1-332-83738-0
PIBN 10172487

This book is a reproduction of an important historical work. Forgotten Books uses
state-of-the-art technology to digitally reconstruct the work, preserving the original format
whilst repairing imperfections present in the aged copy. In rare cases, an imperfection in
the original, such as a blemish or missing page, may be replicated in our edition. We do,
however, repair the vast majority of imperfections successfully; any imperfections that
remain are intentionally left to preserve the state of such historical works.

1 MONTH OF
FREE
READING

at
www.ForgottenBooks.com

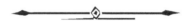

By purchasing this book you are eligible for one month membership to ForgottenBooks.com, giving you unlimited access to our entire collection of over 700,000 titles via our web site and mobile apps.

To claim your free month visit:

www.forgottenbooks.com/free172487

English
Français
Deutsche
Italiano
Español
Português

www.forgottenbooks.com

Mythology Photography **Fiction**
Fishing Christianity **Art** Cooking
Essays Buddhism Freemasonry
Medicine **Biology** Music **Ancient**
Egypt Evolution Carpentry Physics
Dance Geology **Mathematics** Fitness
Shakespeare **Folklore** Yoga Marketing
Confidence Immortality Biographies
Poetry **Psychology** Witchcraft
Electronics Chemistry History **Law**
Accounting **Philosophy** Anthropology
Alchemy Drama Quantum Mechanics
Atheism Sexual Health **Ancient History**
Entrepreneurship Languages Sport
Paleontology Needlework Islam
Metaphysics Investment Archaeology
Parenting Statistics Criminology
Motivational

HEART DISEASE AND ANEURISM IN THE ARMY.

THE CAUSES OF ORIGIN

OF

HEART DISEASE AND ANEURISM

IN THE ARMY:

BY

WILLIAM E. RIORDAN,

Surgeon-Major, Army Medical Department.

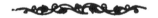

DUBLIN:

FANNIN & CO., 41 GRAFTON-STREET.

LONGMANS, GREEN & CO., LONDON.

1878

11248

PREFACE.

IN presenting this little book to the profession, and more especially those my brother officers to whom the subject is naturally of far more immediate importance and interest, I trust its shortcomings and omissions will be leniently dealt with; for I am living far away from the sources of our knowledge—merely interesting myself by occupying spare moments during the year, while stationed at Port Royal, Jamaica, Barbadoes, and Demerara, where there are no advantages and little opportunities of acquiring information, that would tend to elucidate many points in connection with our subject. Thus thrown very much upon my own resources, I have endeavoured, under these difficulties, to bring the matter forward, and express my views as to the cause of origin of a class of diseases from which the British soldier suffers excessively, and which must be considered as worthy of most serious consideration, both as regard the army and the state.

If it should appear to anyone that I have been rather abrupt in setting aside the opinions of others, while endeavouring clearly and tersely to establish my own views, they may rest assured that no such disrespect was ever intended.

W. E. RIORDAN,
Surgeon-Major.

BRITISH GUIANA,
6th February, 1878.

CONTENTS.

CHAPTER I.

CHAPTER II.

CHAPTER III.

CHAPTER IV.

CHAPTER V.

CHAPTER VI.

CHAPTER VII.

CHAPTER VIII.

DISEASE OF THE HEART AND ANEURISMS IN THE ARMY.

CHAPTER I.

Introduction.—Reference to the amount and peculiarity of diseases of the circulatory system in the army, and supposed causes of origin.—The importance of the subject.—Dr. Hunter's views.—Dr. Maclean's evidence as to the early age disease occurs in the soldier.; the excessive amount of palpitation ; his views, remarks, etc.—Statement of the Pack Committee.—The received idea as to the cause of origin.—Statement from Parkes's *Hygiene*, showing the prevalence of disease in young soldiers, and all arms of the service.—Evidence that there is no diminution in cardiac affections up to date.—Remarks on foregoing.—Opinion expressed that the various conditions in connection with the soldiers' duties are the principal cause of functional derangement of the heart.— Statement from Dr. Fothergill.

THAT sickness should occur to a greater extent among our troops than amongst the civil male population of the soldier's class and age, although the former may be better housed, clad, and fed, is not at all remarkable, when their conditions of service are taken into account, especially such incidental conditions as those in con-nection with tropical service ; and as regards mortality, although from all causes collectively the soldier's mortality is not, as far as we can judge, above that of the civil population, still it appears the soldier ages quicker, gets worn out sooner, and dies comparatively more rapidly as years advance. Moreover, when-ever found incapable of performing further military duties, he is invalided from the service, and "some uncertain addition ought to be made to the mortality on this account."

If affections of the circulatory system were proportionally high

1

among soldiers' diseases, the circumstance could easily be accounted for; but when we find that this class of diseases occurs to an alarming extent, and out of all proportion, among young men who have recently been selected for the service—sound, and as a rule in perfect health—it becomes remarkable, more especially when we find that in these young men it bears a certain peculiarity not observed to any extent in civil life—a certain form of functional derangement of the heart. And as it is these young men also that are most liable to organic diseases of the heart and aneurisms of the aorta, and further, that, contrary to the rule observed in other affections, collectively the death rate from diseases of the circulatory system is highest among young soldiers, so contrary is this to what happens in civil life, it seems strange that such should be the case. And even from these broad facts alone, one might be inclined to think that the cause of the one special affection probably is the same as tends to develop other diseases of the circulatory system. I shall try and couple facts, and bring together evidences, so as to point out that such is really the case ; that the excessive amount of organic heart disease, and the extraordinary prevalence of aortic aneurisms which occur in the service, are due to that functional derangement of the heart which is almost peculiar to the soldier. Now if this alliance between all this class of affections were admitted, or even partially proved, the matter for future investigation would be simplified or brought more to a focus ; for little else would be left to discover, save what it is that disturbs the equilibrium of the circulation in the first instance.

From statistics, and the recorded evidences of the most accurate observers, it may be taken as a fact that palpitation is the chief affection of the circulatory system in the army, and that this functional derangement is characterised by a certain irritability or excitability of the heart's action; and, curiously enough, this disability is found to be almost entirely confined to men subjected to certain regulations or restrictions enforced by military law. Now existing explanations as to the cause of origin of this disability are far from conclusive. They are insufficient to account for the great excess of disease, or the pathological differences that occur between this class of affections in military and in ordinary life. The principal supposable causes are alcohol, tobacco, syphilis, rheumatism, external pressure of dress and accoutrements, exercise or over exertion at irregular and uncertain periods under unfavourable conditions, etc. Of themselves, some of these causes may be considered almost inadmissible; still they all undoubtedly tend to produce disease; but even taken collectively, they appear insufficient satisfactorily to account for the amount and peculiarity or speciality of affections of this class as they exist in the service.

The supposition that external pressure is the cause of origin of so much disease, does not seem to me at all convincing, although ably supported; while other assigned causes, those of a constitutional nature, for instance, are quite inadequate to account for the enormous amount of disease we have. The late Dr. Parkes remarked that the two most common causes of heart disease in the civil population—namely, "rheumatic fever in the young, and renal disease in old persons"—are not acting to any extent in the army.

Supposing the class of diseases under consideration to be preventable, or that the amount could be reduced, since stocks, packs, and cross-belts have been done away with, and the men relieved from carrying as much weight as formerly, and various sanitary reforms introduced, and the Contagious Diseases Act enforced in many garrison towns, there is no reduction of heart affections or aneurisms in the army. This is a point worthy of attention, for together with sanitary reforms, and those changes in dress and accoutrements which have been carried out with the strictest attention to the principles of relieving pressure on important organs and the circulatory system, while other disabilities have diminished considerably, even independent of the zymotic class, there is certainly no equivalent reduction, if any, in the amount of heart affections. Consequently we may search elsewhere for the causes which give rise to these affections. Perhaps they may be more in connection with internal than ex-

1*

ternal influences, or any constitutional defects of the individuals in whom they occur. So we ought to look well to the heart and brain, with all their mutual actions and reactions, in order to discover the source of this irritability of heart, which is "the soldier's complaint."

I believe it originates in the heart itself, and that the exciting cause is displacement of its mechanical arrangements, owing to the sudden alteration of the shape and position of the chest during the setting-up drill of the recruit, and also to the various nervous influences set in action at the same time, by reason of the altered conditions of life to which the recruit is subjected.

Here it may be well to draw attention to the importance of the subject, to ascertain to what extent this class of disease exists in the service, and what the received idea is as to its cause of origin.

Dr. Maclean, writing about diseases of the heart, in the *Army Medical Report* for 1867, says :—" I cannot pass from this subject without doing justice to the memory of a highly meritorious medical officer, the late Staff-Surgeon R. H. Hunter, formerly of the 2nd Queen's Royal Regiment. This officer was the first, as far as I know, to direct attention to the true cause of prevalence of diseases of the heart and great vessels in the army. . . . Dr. Hunter thus expressed his views : 'Ever since I joined the 2nd Queen's at Colaba in 1831, I have been struck with the frequency of cardiac and aortic disease. At first I thought it might be connected with some morbid state of the blood which gave rise to purpura, so frequent at that station; but it afterwards prevailed to an equal extent at Poona, where no such cause could be assigned ; neither does it appear to be altogether connected with rheumatism, though certainly most frequently so, but whether or not rheumatism be the first link in the morbid chain, a more sufficient cause for hastening the progress, I am convinced, is the active duty the soldier undergoes whilst buttoned up in his accoutrements. These, by compressing the neck and chest, obstruct the circulation to such a degree as to excite the heart into inordinate action, and cause great hypertrophy in the strong and muscular, or dilatation in the weak and sickly. Again, in the former, the natural resiliency of the aorta being overcome by the inordinate force of the circulation, that vessel yields, dilates, and finally gives way, giving rise to aneurism."

Ever since this was written, these opinions as to the causation of heart affections and aneurisms seem to have prevailed among medical officers, and many figures and circumstances have from time to time been brought to bear on the subject in support of these views ; yet with all the disease we have, there is not much hypertrophy met with in the army, while aneurisms of the aorta are of very frequent occurrence.

As regards the amount of diseases of the circulatory system which occurs in the service, compared with what has been observed among the male civil population of the soldier's age, for obvious reasons it is not at all easy to arrive at just conclusions ; but from statistics drawn up for the purpose, it may be stated that heart affections are about four or five times, and aneurisms say fifteen times more frequent among our troops. Inspector-General Lawson proved that deaths alone from aortic aneurisms were eleven times more numerous in the army ; and we shall see hereafter that the deaths probably represent but a very small proportion of the disease. To what extent this class of affections exists in the service can more easily and accurately be ascertained, both comparatively as regards other classes of disease, and its relation or connection with other diseases.

In the report referred to, Dr. Maclean states :—"The Royal Victoria Hospital was open for the reception of sick on the 10th of March, 1863. Between that date and the 10th March, 1869, 22,625 invalides have been admitted from abroad, the vast majority being from India. Of this number 1,635 were sent home unfit for duty from disease of the heart." The following remarks from such an authority on this subject are worthy of attention:— "That cases classified as valvular and cardiac disease were for the most part cases of palpitation;" and further, and this, too, is well worthy of note, he says :—"Taking 151 cases of heart disease from our clinical records, 82 were under 30 years of age, and 39 between

30 and 40. It is a notable fact that in only six cases had the patients suffered from acute rheumatism; and again, a very notable fact in the above figures is the early age of the patients affected with both heart disease and aneurism of the aorta. Of the above cases, it appears only 22 had a distinctly recorded history of syphilis, and in only one was there evidence of a gouty diathesis; further, in 72 cases the aortic valves were diseased, and in 54 the mitral."

Here then may be seen the prevalence of the disease, and also to what extent it seems to be developed in India, while attention is directed to the chief peculiarity of these affections as they exist in the service—namely, the extraordinary amount of palpitation. To this I would beg special attention—the early age of men suffering from this affection, as well as from organic disease and aneurisms of the aorta; and although the cardiac valves are remarkably free from disease, when it does occur, we see the aortic are most frequently affected, while the converse holds good in civil life. Naturally; for when the valves are affected by rheumatism, renal, or constitutional diseases, the mitral are more often affected. And here we may notice that it has not escaped his observation to remark on the absence of such diseases in most of the cases. As regards cardiac valvular affections in the army, it is almost quite out of the question that they could be due to constitutional disease; for the cause above all others of these affections is acute rheumatism, producing endocarditis and affecting the mitral valves; and it appears* it rarely manifests itself as an imperfection sufficient in degree to interfere with function until at least middle life.

Dr. Maclean continues :—"I do not think there is much difference of opinion among army medical officers who have enquired carefully into the causation of this large amount of suffering and loss by invaliding. The evidences furnished from this hospital, and the careful enquiries of the Pack Committee, point unequivocally to dress and accoutrements as the active agents in this distressing amount of mischief. The Pack Committee have,

* According to Sir William Jenner.

I believe, solved both the mechanical and physiological problems submitted for their consideration." Again, in the Report for 1870, he says :—"214 cases of heart disease were under treatment during the year : 82 were cases of palpitation. India and other foreign countries furnished 200 of these cases."

While remarking on these figures he writes :—"The allegation, it must be remembered, is not against the knapsack *alone, but against tight clothes and the regulation belts,* which interfere with the mechanism of breathing wherever they are worn. It is obvious that in this costly class of diseases to the military surgeon and to the state prevention is the all-important point. When organic disease of the heart is once established, the case, so far as cure is concerned, is beyond the reach of art—the man becomes at once unfit for military duty, and must as quickly as possible be discharged the service. Much may be done to palliate the disease, to diminish suffering, and to prolong life, and this is daily done by the judicious physician, but for the most part in civil life, to which those thus affected must be relegated. The subject then is well worthy of the closest attention on the part of regimental surgeons, who should narrowly watch the effects of the new system of accoutring the soldier, and should it so happen that, contrary to the expectation of those who have urged the change, no striking diminution in the mortality and invaliding from diseases of the heart and great vessels should result, then the subject should be taken up *de novo* with the view of obtaining a more satisfactory result."

A little further on may be seen that there is no diminution in this class of disease up to the present, and that palpitation is apparently on the increase. I shall now abstract from Mr. Myers's essay,* published in 1870, the conclusions arrived at by the above Committee. "The statement of the medical members of the Committee (appointed by Government, in 1864, to inquire into the subject) as to the mode in which they supposed diseases of the heart to be produced in the army, was as follows :—'During exertion the movements of the chest increase greatly,

* "Alexander" Prize Essay—"Diseases of the Heart among Soldiers.",

deeper breathings are made, the diameter of the chest enlarges in all directions, causing greater expansion of the lungs; the blood flows much more rapidly, and the changes in it and the evolution of carbonic acid are trebled and quadrupled in amount, and the heart acts much more quickly and forcibly. If anything destroys the equilibrium between the powerful action of the heart and the capacity of the lungs to receive the blood propelled into them by the heart, the necessary consequence is an accumulation of blood in the cavities and walls of the heart, which leads to an imperfect action of that organ, and to organic changes in its cavities and walls. . . . The young soldier's ribs and breast-bone, while still soft and pliable, are prevented from proper movements by tight-fitting clothes, and by the straps of accoutrements and packs. Of these the cross-belt, bearing the pouch, is the most objectionable, as it passes across the chest, and impedes the movement forward of the breast-bone. The waist-belt, also, if too tight, hinders the expansion of the lower ribs. The knapsack straps are less hurtful in this way; but they also press to some extent on the collar-bone and first ribs. It will be seen, therefore, that there is a combination of actions all leading to the same result. The mature soldier, with his bones all formed, and his muscles full-grown and strong, may perhaps bear these constrictions without injury; but not so the young man. It is probable, however, that more or less injury is done to all.' "

Here, after stating the phenomena observed during exertion in the respiratory and circulatory process, it is stated that if *anything* destroys the equilibrium of the process it leads to imperfect action of the heart, and organic changes in its cavities and walls ; and as the young soldier's chest is pliable, tight fitting clothes and belts will interfere with the process; hence I suppose they conclude that exertion taken under such unfavourable conditions was the cause of all excess of heart disease in the army ; and this still appears to be the received idea. Yet as we look into the matter we shall see that there are very many other things acting on the heart of the young soldier liable to upset its equilibrium. Organic changes in the heart are not of very remarkable frequency in the army, and since the recommenda- tions founded on the above views have been carried out, statis- tics do not show any diminution of cardiac affections, while, if anything, they are, compared with home service, more prevalent in India, where there is relaxation without any restrictions to the chest, and no exertion taken under such unfavourable conditions.

Parkes, in his *Practical Hygiene*, writes:—"The fact that dis- eases of the circulatory system rank second as causes of death in the army at home, may well surprise us. It is marked in all arms—as much in the artillery and cavalry as in the infantry. The ratio per 1,000 of strength for the last five years (1867-'71) for all diseases of the organs of circulation is 1.462, and in these years, out of every 100 deaths, no less than 16·7 were from dis- eases of the heart and vessels. In addition there is a large amount of invaliding from this cause. . . These numbers are higher than those of the nine years 1859-'67, when the mortal- ity from circulatory diseases was only ·908 per 1,000 of strength, and the percentage on the total deaths was nine."

When considered from what cause these diseases are supposed to originate, it seems curious that they occur almost equally in the different arms of the service ; for the men are differently dressed, armed, accoutred, and employed.

The cavalry wear a sword belt, and light shoulder belt, and no pack, the horse carries the valise; lancers wear sword belts only ; and drivers in the artillery are unarmed men ; while of latter years, with all the improvements in dress and accoutre- ments, the death rate from diseases of the circulatory system has actually increased from 9 to 16·7 per cent., a circumstance most probably due to the reduced strength of regiments, which tends to throw more strain on its component parts; while autumn manœuvres and rapidity of movements all tend to develop dis- ease and render it more fatal. There are yet other causes that may give rise to this increased amount of disease ; for instance, the rapidity with which recruits are put through their drill of

late years, the amount they have to learn, and the degree of
smartness required of them.   Formerly a recruit was given four
or five months to pass through his course of instruction.   The
thing was done quietly.   The demand for men with the colours
was not so great ; but now the setting-up drill is done under high
pressure ; and I hope to be able to point out, that in recruits'
drill, by suddenly altering the shape of the chest and thereby displacing the arrangements of the heart and great vessels, we will
discover the principal mechanical cause which disturbs the
equilibrium of the circulatory process.

Again, soldiers, especially young men, seem to pass through
more prison life of late years.   Now, by reason of living under
discipline or certain rules or restrictions enforced by military
law, even independent of those punishments awarded by commanding officers and carried out regimentally, soldiers are further
subjected to the deleterious influences of prison regime to a far
greater extent than the civil community of their class ; and here
we may find another cause of development of cardiac affections.

To bring the matter up to date—taking the last published
Army Medical Report, the *Blue Book* for 1874, it may be seen
that 16·8 per 1,000 of the admissions to hospital at home were
from diseases of the circulatory system, being an increase on
the previous five years ; and during this year, for the same
class of diseases, 321 men were invalided from India, and it is
stated :—" In this year, as compared with 1873, the invaliding
due to diseases of the circulatory system is ·34 per 1,000 in excess : the proportion of one disease in the order, *Palpitation*, is
in a ratio of ·95 per 1,000 in excess of that of the previous years."

In the *Army Medical Report* for 1875, just received by me, I
find, although diseases of the circulatory system in the army
serving in the United Kingdom are more prevalent than during
the previous year, with respect to palpitation it seems an exceptional year ; for we read at page 17 :—" The point of most interest
in connection with diseases of this order is the evidence of arrest
of the hitherto progressive rise in the ratio of admissions for
palpitation. . . .   The decrease of ·1 per 1,000 on the

corresponding rates of 1874." The number of civil practitioners employed may account for this, for men unaccustomed to meet with this special affection and its distressing symptoms are more likely than military men to diagnose it as organic disease. Again, at page 25, we read : "Admissions for functional diseases of the heart are in the following proportions :—Dragoons, 6·64 ; Royal Artillery, 7·22 ; Foot Guards, 3·58 ; and Infantry, 7·76 per 1,000 men. Compared with the preceding year, the proportion for Foot Guards shows an increase of 2·85 per 1,000 men. No admissions for palpitation took place in Household Cavalry in either year." What the internal economy of the Household Cavalry is, or how discipline is applied and enforced, I do not know, but suspect their system is different from that of the rank and file of the army. In this year also may be seen that 343 men were invalided from India on account of the same group of diseases ; and we find among this increased number sent home, 94 men were sent from Bengal on account of palpitation, for which disability 29 were also invalided from Madras. I can find nothing in this Report that could induce me to alter what has been already written, or add any new matter.

Here then we see the great importance of this subject. It is indeed well worthy of our closest attention. We also see that palpitation is the principal affection in this class of disease to which the soldier is particularly liable, and after the recommendations made by the Committee of 1864—to relieve, as far as possible, all undue pressure—have been carried out and tried for years, the disease has not diminished in the service. From this fact alone, and without further consideration, one might be almost inclined to conclude that they have not discovered the true cause of origin of these affections ; or at any rate, as before remarked, supposing the cause to be avoidable, proper remedies for its prevention or removal have not been taken ; for with all our tact and knowledge, the disease is actually increasing. Thus I think the time has come to investigate the matter *de novo*, for there are probably other and more subtle causes at work to account for all this loss to the state, and human suffering, than

mere mechanical obstruction to the respiratory process or impeded circulation. There is, be it observed, an increase in the
amount of palpitation. This may, perchance, be only an apparent
increase. For instance, on account of the great expense incurred
by invaliding, presidents of boards required at one time strong
cases to be made out before sending men home, and this may
account for many of the apparent errors in diagnoses noticed by
Dr. Maclean at Netley, where cases classed as valvular and cardiac
disease were for the most part cases of palpitation ; and now it
appears more thoroughly understood that mere functional derangement is quite sufficient to incapacitate men from further
military duties.

I think I am right in saying, a considerable amount of palpitation yet exists which does not find its way into statistics. It
is without recognition, and included under other headings even
independent of the circulatory system, such as general debility,
dyspepsia, etc.

Before proceeding to investigate the matter, in order to ascertain how far various causes may be likely to give rise to the
functional or nervous derangement included in the statistical
returns under the head of palpitation, perhaps it would be well
to state more fully my belief that it is of a dynamic nature, and
not of a secondary nature brought on through any constitutional
disease of poisonous influences, or any effort of the heart to overcome obstruction to the circulation.

Anything that displaces the heart or alters its position in the
chest, and its relation or connection with other organs, or unduly
disturbs the nervous centres, or interferes with the transmission
of nerve-force to the heart, will excite its irritability. We shall
see that in the soldier, and especially in those newly joined, by
reason of their being subjected to discipline and the anxieties
attendant on military duties, there is a constant nervous strain.
To be at all times ready for emergencies, to be subjected to many
masters, to be constantly under supervision or restraint, to live by
the clock, to move by bugle call, to be always up to time, produces
a never-ceasing strain on the nervous centres, which tends to

nervous exhaustion. If the duties are but imperfectly understood, the strain is all the greater; while on parade, or at other times during the day, all manifestation of the emotions likely to arise from mental disturbance, anxieties, worry, or annoyances, are strictly forbidden, either by word or gesture. Thus the soldier is subjected to the internal pressure of pent-up feelings, and I hope to bring evidence to show how directly all these conditions react on the heart.

"It is possible there may exist conditions essentially nervous, when a derangement of the balance of nerve-supply to the heart, a disturbance of the balance existing between the cardiac ganglia of the sympathetic, and the inhibitory action of the pneumogastric, may occasion palpitation; but of these conditions we do not yet know anything clinically. . . Increasing knowledge of the pathological conditions, and the advance of our acquaintance with the mode of action of disordered functions, are shedding much light on what have been hitherto obscure cardiac derangements."—*Fothergill.*

CHAPTER II.

Showing the probable connection between the majority of diseases of the circulatory system in the army.—Evidences of the nature of the functional derangement of the heart met with among troops.—Dr. Henry Hartshorne's observations on this affection in the army of the United States of America.—Remarks on muscular and nervous exhaustion of heart.—Evidences of the similarity of what occurs among our troops.—The Committee's Report.—Mr. Myers's views as to the causation of disease.—The age of our recruits.—Sphygmographic tracings of the pulse in functional derangement.—Note from Parkes.—Some pathological differences and peculiarities in soldiers' diseases compared with what occurs in civil life.—Remarks, etc.

Now taking some evidence in connection with the symptoms recorded from clinical observations of that rather obscure cardiac derangement met with among troops, they may shed a little light on the subject, and we shall see that other armies are subject to an affection similar to that which pervades our own. Dr. Henry Hartshorne, writing in 1864 on heart disease in the army of the United States of America [*Half-Yearly Abstract of Medical Sciences*, vol. xl.], remarks on what he calls muscular exhaustion of the heart, differing from ordinary palpitation; and after referring to dilatation and hypertrophy, says—(and to the following I would direct special attention) :—"Yet the majority of heart diseases under my observation were not cases of either form of enlargement of the heart. . . The symptoms were rapidity with comparative feebleness of pulse, while the patient was at rest; great acceleration of the heart's movements on the slightest exertion. An impulse in proportion to its acceleration was rather below than above the normal average force, and was sudden and short, not heaving. . . These cases occurred in men who went through the privations of the Potomac campaign, and were anæmic, but when the anæmia was removed, the disability still remained. . . The physical signs observed in the majority of these cases were as follows : no extension of dullness on percussion beyond the usual limits, and sometimes even less than natural; impulse without unusual force, and especially deficient relatively to its acceleration, having also a short although hardly a jerking movement, but quite different from the heaving movements of concentric hypertrophy, and not lifting the ear or stethoscope so much even as transient functional palpitation ; sounds of the heart free from murmur in almost all cases. There was present, however, a comparative deficiency in duration and loudness in the first sound, and a proximation to it in the character of the second sound."

This condition, if I understand him correctly, was known at the hospital as the " trotting heart," and he considered it brought on by " prolonged exertion, privation of rest, deficient food, bad water, and malaria." He says, " the only supposable hypotheses in regard to the affection under consideration are : 1st. A symptom of general anaemia ; 2nd. A scorbutic symptom ; 3rd. A variety of palpitation due to alcohol, tobacco, or coffee."

Here then is a most admirable description, almost quite typical of the phenomena observed in the irritable or excitable heart found so frequently among our troops ; but as our men are not subjected to the same privations as the Americans were, the explanation as to its causation will not hold good for us; neither will the supposable hypotheses apply in our case; so we must look elsewhere, for all these are of so incidental a nature that they may be left out of the calculation, as quite insufficient to account for the excessive amount of disease we have. The disease, observe, was without hypertrophy; this point seems to be particularly noted, the impulse was short, and neither was there the long, irregular systole, slow and often intermittent, so often observed in that variety of palpitation which results from such poisons as alcohol or tobacco; the irregularity in such cases being probably correctly accounted for by the power disturbing the balance of nerve-force supplying the cardiac ganglia acting on some· more than on others. There is no mention made of the effects of clothing in these cases : perhaps little time was spent in tailoring to a tight fit. Neither is there any reference to the age of the men affected. Probably they were men, the so-called bone and sinew of the country or other countries, hurriedly drilled under great excitement, conducted to the front, and subjected to a strictly enforced discipline. Such causes are capable of laying the foundation of diseases. They produce a constant nervous strain, liable to be followed by nervous exhaustion of the heart, hastened or developed under the conditions in which the men were subsequently placed ; and this is pretty much the case with our soldiers in India, from whence we receive home so very many invalids similarly affected, for there climatic influences assist in its development.

Fatigues following exertion, as they are preceded by increased heart's action, may be said to produce muscular exhaustion of that organ, or in so marked a manner develop latent disability as to lead to the belief that over or prolonged exertion under unfavourable mechanical conditions was the cause of the excessive amount of disease in our army. But we must bear well in mind that over-excitement, or prolonged nervous tension, or causes of any description that have a depressing influence on the nervous centres, will directly produce nervous exhaustion of the heart. Irritability is of a nervous nature, and in all instances nervous exhaustion seems preferable to muscular exhaustion of the heart ; for the vital agency that gives power of action to the muscles is nervous, and it is this agency that is affected in the first instance, whether through poison, fatigue, or mental influences. The functional derangement of the muscle fibre is secondary, and merely the manifestation of the nervous derangement. We shall refer to this point again.

Now by taking some evidences of the affection observed among our troops it may be seen how very closely the symptoms resemble what have been observed in the American army ; so much so, that they must be considered as the same affection, as indeed they are.

I shall frequently have occasion to quote Mr. Myers's essay, from which I hope to derive much valuable assistance; for as well as containing most reliable information—information it would be impossible for me otherwise to obtain—it is also the best exposition of the views entertained by those who have had the greatest facilities for studying the subject.

At page 38 he accounts for the origin of purely functional derangement in our service, as follows. At the age of the recruit, the protecting case of the heart and lungs has not sufficiently ossified to resist the external pressure to which the chest is subjected, and the heart has not at this age attained its full growth; for, according to Boyd, its average weight in males from 14 to 20 years of age is 7·61 ounces, and from 20 to 30 years of age 10·96 ounces, and therefore this organ, unable to cope with the difficulties suddenly imposed upon it, takes on an irritability or excitability of action which gradually becomes more apparent as the cause is continued; or after a time, owing to the normal growth of the heart, this functional derangement may subside in some cases. On examination, at this time, percussion reveals little or no increase of cardiac dullness; the sounds of the heart are short and abrupt, the second being abnormally distinct; the apex beat is visible below the left nipple, and the pulse is small and very rapid. The Committee to whom I have already referred, in drawing attention to this condition, stated:—"The special heart disease from which the young soldier suffers is not, we are informed, disease of the valves, but an extreme excitability of the heart, combined with some, but not great, enlargement. During rest, a heart of this kind beats easily, but on the least exertion, its action becomes irregular, and the man becomes breathless." "The heart at this time not being fully developed, its hypertrophy cannot be easily recognized, and I am inclined to think that this permanent irritability is much dependent on the partial absence of hypertrophy; dilatation of one or more cavities, however, ere long becomes apparent."

Here then is a description which shows the similarity of the affection so well known in our army to that which was observed by Dr. H. Hartshorne; yet they are supposed to originate from very different causes. I do not consider the average size of the heart of lads between 14 and 20 years of age admissible as an argument that our recruits have comparatively weak or small hearts, for they are not of such tender years. And it must be remembered that they are frequently drilled without any restrictions to the chest. Of the 30,557 recruits passed into the service in 1874, 25,157 were from 18 to 23 years of age; and more than twice as many came in between 22 and 23 as between 17 and 18; under 17 only a few boys are taken by special authority. But admitting the point for a moment—although these figures evidently show that it rests on a false basis—the weaker and smaller the heart, the less chance there is of its injuring the aorta. Here is a difficulty that might be overcome by again admitting the idea that partial hypertrophy exists extensively, and further, that this partial hypertrophy is the cause of permanent irritability. I shall refer to this hereafter when considering the causation of aneurisms; but as far as I know, this is the only explanation given as to the manner in which external pressure creates palpitation of an irritative type, and permanently establishes the disability.

I cannot pass from these evidences as to this special affection, even at the risk of being tedious in quoting authorities on a subject generally so well known to army medical officers, without referring to a foot note in the last edition of Parkes's *Hygiene*. He writes :—" The cardiac diseases are of the most varied kind. I have seen at Netley, in Dr. Maclean's wards, in one hour in the summer, when the hospital is full, almost all the combinations of heart affections. It has appeared to me that if anything gives the tendency to heart affections, then the dress and the accoutrements come in as accessory causes, and prevent all chance of cure. In some cases there is no valvular disease, and not much hypertrophy of the heart, but a singular excitability ; so that the heart beats frightfully quick on the least exertion."

Although every variety and all combinations of heart affections exist in the service, there is nothing as regards their frequency of occurrence to arrest our attention, in comparison with that of functional or nervous derangement. So we shall at present deal with it, in order if possible to discover what it is that gives rise to this affection—a form of palpitation which is exemplified in a quick, short muscular effort, with a somewhat jerking action. This marks the first sound of the heart, and conveys a throbbing tremor to the large arteries, with a somewhat feeble pulse at the wrist, for the amount of force expended at the heart. This comparative feebleness of the pulse I think due to the small amount of blood sent forward at each impulse of the heart; for it is highly probable the left ventricle contracts in its excited state when insufficiently filled. Now this will explain most of the foregoing phenomena, and will also satisfactorily account for the diastolic wave observed in the pulse in these cases, and which is said to be characteristic of functional derangement of this description. Be it observed, the venous circulation in these instances is quiet. There is no severe muscular exertion required to produce the symptoms, no call for increased blood being circulated, nor any flushing of the face to indicate increased supply of blood to the system. Hurry of the respiration to any notable extent is of very rare occurrence, and in these cases, the strength of the muscle soon fails, and the individual as a rule becomes weak and faint. I need not dwell on symptoms which are only too well known in our service ; but would draw attention to this point especially, as it is thus that the increased action, sending only a small quantity of blood into the aorta, can go on for years without causing hypertrophy ; and as a physical sign Dr. Hartshorne observed, in the majority of his cases, there was no extension of dullness beyond the usual limits and *sometimes being even less than natural* in these latter instances, is it not highly probable the heart remained in a semi-contracted state through nervous irritability, and never properly expanded to receive a due amount of blood. Thus the moment any slight exertion is taken, requiring the circulation of more blood than usual, in order to supply the want a heart in this condition *must* beat inordinately quick. The abnormal quickness with which the heart beats on the least exertion in very

2*

many instances is well known to us, although this condition of
heart, as we shall see, is probably brought on by a variety of
causes acting with one tendency.   Yet when the condition is
established as a defect, it is the *habit* acquired by palpitation,
the frequently-recurring increased heart's action, which induces
nerve-force, once liberated, to be expended at the heart, for
nerve-force prefers to flow along those channels which are the
most customary route through which it has been transmitted.
Thus habit alone may cause a recurrence of the derangement,
although at the time there is but little exertion taken to call
for increased heart's action.   The irritability of the heart,
causing its contractions to come quick and vigorous, produces
a stretching and expansion of the large arteries, and there
are few muscular fibres in their coats to enable them to resist
or guard against this effect ; thus they throb as they receive
the jet of blood ; but the instant the short, forcible expansive
pressure of the blood, propelled by the excited or uncontrolled
heart, acting, it may be, through its own inherent irritability,
is taken off, the arteries contract to the same calibre as they
were previously to being dilated, and being elastic, with a
similar degree of force to that which caused their expansion.
This throws back the blood, which had not sufficient time to
be distributed, with great force on the aortic valves, and thus,
closing them with a bang, produces the loud second sound
observed in these cases.   A small quantity of blood being
squirted well and smartly into the aorta, the recoil will be all
the more forcible, and having space left to flow back against the
valves, it gives an abnormally marked depression to the tidal
wave—each wave as it were being divided instead of bearing a
mere ripple from the vibration of the valves and tension of the
vessels.   When the phenomenon thus produced is projected as
far as the radial pulse, it may be so modified as to be of little
value in determining the original physical cause that produces
the sphygmographic tracings, as compared with observations
taken from arteries springing from the aorta.   By the time the
impulse or vibration of the tidal wave has been transmitted

to the wrist, it has traversed tubings supplied with muscles, which can be independently affected by nervous agency, and this may give rise to modifications due to contraction or expansion of their calibre, for it appears muscular fibres do actually elongate by innervation ; but this inherent power of producing throbbings is quite different from the elastic swellings due to mechanical causes. Yet, however modified cases may be, Mr. Myers (page 40) says of those cases examined by him— " more or less marked dicrotism was present in each specimen ;" and he considers it characteristic of functional derangement, and agrees with those who believe it to be owing to the recoil of blood against the valves, which is undoubtedly the case.

Now the next point is, why is the recoil so peculiar as to give rise to this diagnostic sign?—why does it not occur in hypertrophy for instance ? The origin of this dip in the pulse wave may be accounted for, not as a consequence of the yieldingness of the arteries, but only on account of the amount of blood sent forward at each systole of the ventricles. In hypertrophy we have extreme tension of the arteries, and they may be quite as yielding as in cases of mere functional derangement; but owing to the column of blood sent forward filling up the entire artery, the expansion is not of short duration ; for they cannot recover their pre-systolic calibre until the blood is distributed. Considering the arteries are passive agents in both instances, and not regarding elasticity as a vital process, the rapidity or short duration of their expansion has no influence over their contraction, nor can it effect the abruptness with which the valves are closed by the returning blood. It is the quantity of blood, together with the distance it is shot clear of the valves, by allowing room for recoil, that gives a pause in the pulse wave, and again a shock to the column of blood, and thus makes the diastolic wave, which is most apparent when the artery has lost its tone. The recoil in cases of hypertrophy resulting from any cause, from obstruction say, being from a greater column of fluid, may be as forcible, or possibly even more so; but for want of space, the artery being filled, it cannot flop back against the valves; hence there is no such marked wave, no abnormally loud second sound described as re-sembling the first.

I do not believe that any effort of the heart to carry on its own vital functions, under mechanical obstruction to the free flow of blood, aortic, or other obstruction, or that arising through abnormal density of the blood or regurgitation through disease of the aortic valves, which is equivalent to obstruction, would give rise to the same train of phenomena as occur in the soldier's heart, and hypertrophy or dilatation; organic disease would quickly be established, while the absence of organic disease, after years of this derangement, has been frequently remarked. The symptoms and evidences are too strong facts to admit the sup-position that hypertrophy exists to any extent. If to overcome resistance was the object sought, by an effort of nature the contrac-tion of the ventricles would be abnormally prolonged, instead of short and quick. It is in order to overcome resistance that the systole of the ventricles is so much longer than that of the auricles; again, where there is hypertrophy, the patient scarcely knows there is anything wrong; but in the soldier's complaint the symptoms are most severe and distressing.

From whatever cause the aortic valves perform their functions imperfectly, hypertrophy or dilatation will result. Now it has been remarked as strange that cases of hypertrophy frequently occur in the army without disease of these valves. Of another peculiarity, Mr. Myers, after referring to two typical cases under his observation, says :—" These cases represent a form of disease which is rarely found in the civil population, but which I believe is by no means uncommon in the army—viz., disease of the aor-tic valves, and of these valves only, secondary to hypertrophy of the left ventricle, and without any known history of disease to account for this hypertrophy; whereas, in the civil population, disease of the aortic valves alone is uncommon, as already shown; and when existing is found to precede, and not to follow the hypertrophy."

Now without there being any abnormal check to the circula-tion, the circumstance of hypertrophy occurring, either without or preceding the valvular affection, can be easily explained, and cases of this description rather strengthen my views, that organic disease is for the most part due to the irritability of the heart ; for when the elasticity of the aorta becomes worn out by the too frequent over-stretching to which the vessel is subjected, it becomes flaccid, and thus the valves are not closed by the return of blood—they remain open for a short period after the stroke of the ventricle ; consequently the heart, in addition to the blood brought by the venous circulation, is obliged to pump what drips back into the aorta again, and this increased work leads to hypertrophy or may be dilatation, without disease of the valves. It is the irritability of the heart, by destroying the elasticity of the aorta, prevents its squeezing back the blood on the valves, and by rushing into the sinuses behind them shut them up. Thus their functions are imperfectly performed, through no fault of theirs, and after death they are found in a normal condition, or may be somewhat thickened, on account of the unusual flapping and friction to which they were subjected during the functional disease from which the organic proceeded.

From the above cause, some fibres of the aorta generally lose their elasticity before others, and this produces a roughness in the lining membrane which may lead to an error in diagnosis, even with a most practised ear. Of course the same may result from hypertrophy. Again anæmia from climate, combined with splenic and liver enlargements, by interfering with the heart, may give rise to abnormal sounds; still the disease is functional as far as the heart is concerned, and it is its own dynamic powers that are upset through mechanical interference and poisonous influences giving rise to perverted innervation, or disturbing the balance of nerve-force at the heart.

This seems to be the case with many men invalided in India for England, suffering from derangement of the heart. Of course when they arrive at Bombay, some months later, after a march down country, with all the cheering prospects of getting home, or still later on at Netley, after a sea voyage, with rest and relaxation from military duty—that fertile source of this derangement

—all symptoms of the disability may have disappeared. The heart then has regained the position from which it was displaced and the nervous centres have recovered their tone. Furthermore, when the artery has its functions impaired, it is liable to become affected with some form of degeneration or decay, and when abrasions of the lining membrane are once formed in subjects afflicted with constitutional syphilis, they may take on a syphilitic character, and so lead to the belief that the syphilitic virus was the original cause of the disability. But aortic aneurisms, occurring, as they do occur in the service, without hypertrophy or any pathological sign of disease in the vessel, can only be accounted for by considering the starting point to be mere functional derangement.

Having referred to the amount of disease of the circulatory system, which in itself shows the importance of the subject, and having exemplified the phenomena usually observed in the heart affections to which soldiers are particularly liable, and enumerated to some extent the circumstances or causes that are supposed to give rise to the train of symptoms observed both in our army and that of the United States of America, attention was drawn to the circumstance that the excess of organic disease and aneurism may be brought about solely by one cause—namely, the irritability of the heart ; for *without the respiratory or circulatory process being impeded in any way*, it can destroy the elasticity of the aorta, and thus, by rendering it unable to contract, the valves are not closed in sufficient time by the returning blood to prevent some dripping back into the ventricle; and this increased quantity to be rejected causes organic disease, without disease of the valves ; or in other instances it may so occur that the aorta being injured, takes on some form of degeneration, and aneurisms follow. Thus it is the different causes of origin which give rise to the pathological differences and peculiarities that exist in the organic heart disease of the army, as compared with what occurs in civil life.

Here then I have tried to connect all heart affections in the service with one another, believing that by far the greater proportion of them proceed from one source ; and these views are further strengthened by the circumstance of the early age at which both functional and organic disease, and also aneurisms, arise, as well as by the late Dr. Parkes's remarks, which are at all times worthy of our utmost attention—"That whatever the cause of the preponderance of disease of the circulatory system in the army may be, it is probable they produce both the cardiac and arterial disease."

CHAPTER III.

Referring to the physical and mental condition of the recruit previous to enlistment.—The classes of men who are entering the service.—The drill instructor's ideas of typical man.—Further proof from Parkes of the quickness with which disease is brought on after enlistment.— The effects of habit in developing muscle, ligament, and bone, and producing certain condition of the frame.—Manual labour brings about a formation of body unfavourable to that erectness of carriage and freedom of movement required in the service.—The effects of changing the inherited or acquired shape of the chest.—Alteration of acquired deformity, by displacing the heart, causes palpitation.—Statement from Dr. Walshe, showing the ease with which the heart can be displaced.

THIS point being so far established, it may be well to introduce the "raw material," not the recruit, as is generally done, but what the recruit is made of; for we must bear well in mind his natural hereditary shapes, and physical and mental conditions, and all his connections and surroundings; before arriving at conclusions, we must compare his former life with the altered conditions of life to which he is subjected, the rapid alteration of his natural formation, and those regulation or incidental circumstances involved in his new career. These things must be considered, for they all bear on the subject, before we can hope to discover the cause of origin of the functional derangement which is the foundation of all excess of heart disease and aneurisms in the army.

The classes of the community from which we derive our best material, are the farm-labourers, ploughmen, or other inhabitants of our rural districts. These people supply undoubtedly the physically best and least vicious recruits; but by reason of their employments they are round shouldered or backed, or otherwise badly set-up men; while, taking trades and other occupations, by reason of their employments—as tailors, shoemakers, weavers, or workers in harder materials—their offspring have either acquired in their own persons, or inherited by reason of the manual labour of their forefathers, certain physical conditions, forms, and shapes necessary for such pursuits as these people follow in civil life ; but the forms thus conferred give them a loutish appearance and awkward carriage, which, be it observed, is perfectly natural to the individual, although quite at variance with our ideas of a smart, soldierlike bearing.

Of the 30,557 recruits inspected in 1874, as may be seen by the last published *Army Medical Report*, group No. 1, labourers, husbandmen, and servants, furnished 18,917, or more than half; group 2; manufacturing artizans, 3,558 ; group 3, mechanics employed in occupations favourable to physical development, 5,391. Now of the entire number only 1,742 were under 18 years of age ; so judging from these three principal groups, the material could not be very soft and pliable; and it is almost out of the question that these individuals could be easily affected by the pressure of the improved dress and accoutrements worn by our soldiers, so soon after joining ; and I will endeavour to point out that, in all probability, where belts press on the upper portion of the chest, that part becomes consolidated at a comparatively early age in the recruit's class.

Now mark this point. The service receives men in their natural state, with certain shapes and forms ; in good health, with all their natural functions, and the circulatory system in perfect order ; and what is done? Why, we promptly set to work to change them into an ideal conformation.

Here let us suppose the drill-sergeant's idea of the natural upright position of man, which exalts him above the brute creation, is that of a soldier at attention, with his chest thrown forward and upward, head erect, back flat, and feet at an angle of forty-five degrees, and that all his movements should be conducted with as close a proximation to this bearing as locomotion will permit. What a sad falling off from this typical standard comes under his observation daily; how he must fancy the human race degenerating, and what anxiety and heart-breaking work to mould them into proper shapes ! Moreover, the older the individual, the less pliable are his bony structures, as they are ossifying into their hereditary curvings, and the vessels settling down into their natural groovings.

Dr. Parkes writes, page 575—"The production of diseases of the circulatory organs begins very early in the military career. In 1860-'62, I calculated out the causes of invaliding in 6,856 men. Of these 1,014 were under two years' service. In the whole number the percentage of heart and vessel disease, as the cause of the invaliding, was 7·7. Among the men under two years' service it was 14·23 per cent. As these men had presumably healthy hearts when they enlisted, the effect both of the military life in producing diseases of the circulatory organs, and the greater suffering from it of young soldiers, seems certain. The statistics of the Knapsack Committee Report confirm this." Here then it is undoubtedly very soon after the recruit joins that his heart gets acted on, and we need no further proof of the quickness with which disease is brought about. I think we shall find it is induced or created during that period after the man is sworn in, when brought under discipline and being instructed and first taught subordination.

Habitually exercising certain muscles will develop them, and their action will modifiy, enlarge, and harden bony structures, so that they may be capable of supporting their action. This can be acquired in an individual; or if similar conditions are long continued in a class, the speciality becomes inherited. It is scarcely worth while giving examples of these well-known principles. External muscles become visibly developed, and in certain trades internal muscles also; such has been remarked of the psoas in top-sawers. The heart also, under increased exertion, becomes remarkably developed, for it is not under control of the will, and has to work without rest : the pause, while filling, is not rest. Again, in countries where the inhabitants are accustomed to carry weights on their heads or shoulders, it is surprising with what ease they can do so, as the class of muscles that

preserve the balance are developed, and this custom is supposed
to give an upright bearing to the people of an entire country.
The spine supports the weight, but the muscles and ligaments
support the spine, otherwise the natural curvings would be increased. Among tribes in the Himalayas, it may be noticed how
much better the muscles of the lower extremities are developed, in
comparison with those of the upper, or with those of the inhabitants of the plains. No doubt this natural conformation is inherited by reason of their having so much uphill work, and
being obliged to carry their own goods and chattles over moun-
tain paths, where no baggage animals, save sheep and goats, could
travel—the load for these quadrupeds is 20 lbs. In the second
place, left-handed men, as a rule, especially in the labouring
classes, have got the spine curved towards that side, and by
reason of this the shoulder is carried higher than the right.
This looks awkward but is quite natural to the individual,
yet it gives a good deal of trouble to the drill-sergeant to
reduce this deformity to the correct level. It occurs to me
the reason of this curving of the spine may be thus accounted
for. The human race are a right-handed race all the world
over, and to preserve symmetry, the muscles and ligaments
of the opposite side are prepared to resist right-hand influence; but when the anomaly of a left-hand comes into play,
it upsets nature by taking her aback, and the opposite side, not
being prepared for the imposition, is turned over. Thus, muscles and ligaments are developed, and as regards bone in the
various trades or occupations in the three principal groups from
which our recruits are obtained, muscles alter by their action the
bony frame-work of the chest, and the lungs, the heart, and
great vessels adapt themselves to carry on their functions under
these altered conditions of the frame.

Causes acting with the same tendency for generations, will
develop certain shapes and conditions. Now, manual labour,
among those whose occupations are considered favourable to
physical development — miners, navvies, ground workers in
general, various trades, and sailors, for most part work in a

bent or stooping position, quite different from soldiers. Thus there is a tendency to stoop, and their arms becoming very heavy by reason of their muscular and bony development, they naturally get round-shouldered or backed, with the blade bones wide apart, and the clavicles short, strong, and curved. The general aspect and bony framework of the chest has undergone changes not in accordance with sculptural symmetry. Moreover, by reason of the position in which they work, the abdominal viscera are kept close up to the diaphragm, so that the lower ribs become expanded, while the upper are fixed, to grant a fulcrum or support to the powerful pectoral muscles. Consequently this portion is not very movable, and most probably, in this situation the temporary cartilages become ossified at an early age. From a similar cause (muscular development), in women accustomed to field work, the pelvis becomes consolidated at an early age. I remember having heard a professor of midwifery say that by looking at the hands of women who came to a lying-in hospital from the country, he could pronounce on a tedious or difficult labour.

Here then the shape of the recruit on enlistment is either acquired or inherited by long habit, and is perfectly natural to the individual as a specimen of his class ; and the clumsy movements conferred by reason of his shape, and long use or disuse of certain muscles, gives him an awkward gait. Where a more general and greater variety of muscular movements take place, without speciality, as in the officer class, there is more symmetry; so that, if officers were dressed exactly like their men, their movements or action would distinguish them, even at a distance. It is the shape, and not muscular development, that gives the action to horse and man; but the point is that muscular action long continued can confer, modify, or alter the shape of the bony framework, and the great difficulty with the recruit is to so change his shape, that by the end of a month or six weeks his movements will be perfect, and in accordance with those laid down by regulation. It is this remodelling or improving on nature—warping her into a typical standard, and thereby sud-

denly altering the shape and position of the chest—that in
very many instances upsets the equilibrium of the circulatory
process.

Now from what has just been stated, is it not highly probable
that the ligaments are strengthened, the temporary cartilages
ossified, and the upper portion of the chest consolidated, at a
comparatively early age in the recruit's class, on account of the
muscular development of the upper extremities ? Consequently
the recruit is better prepared to resist pressure on this portion of
his chest, than at first anticipated. I have already drawn attention to the mature age of the men we are getting.

Cases of acquired deformity of the chest give very good proof
of palpitation being caused by the heart being interfered with.
In some trades, such as shoemakers and coopers, external pressure from the last or stave gives an acquired deformity to the
breast bone; but, as the change is gradual, the heart and arteries
manage to perform their functions naturally: there is no disease.
But if such men were passed into the service, they would not
get through their preliminary drill without developing the irritable heart. I have seen some examples of this. It is generally
well known, and strict injunctions have been given not to pass
such men into the service, although perfectly sound. The last
example of this sort I have seen was in an artillery recruit at
Newbridge. Three of his ribs were depressed since childhood,
about the region of the heart.

The reason why these imperfections render men practically un-
suitable, is that the position drill to which they are subjected, by
altering the shape of the chest, *displaces* the heart. Observe, in
these instances, the heart has not previously been displaced—
although unable to occupy the normal position, it has adapted
itself to circumstances; but when suddenly dislocated, so to
speak, its functions are interfered with, and its action, being
interrupted, becomes irritable and irregular. Where there is deformity, the heart has not the same amount of space left, to carry
on its functions under altered circumstances.

In evidence of the ease with which the heart can be displaced

Dr. Walshe writes :—"The heart, situated in the lower part of the anterior mediastinum, is held *in situ* directly by the great vessels, arterial and venous, and indirectly through the pericardium by the diaphragm. These attachments, fixing the base only of the heart, permit free play of the general mass, which in point of fact hangs loosely in the pericardial sac. This looseness of attachment, and this freedom of movement—essential to the physiological well-being of the organ—entails a specific inconvenience, in the extreme facility with which the heart, in this respect almost rivalling the uterus, undergoes various displacements."

CHAPTER IV.

Conditions imposed by the service, and the mechanical and mental influences which produce disease.—Note the first conditions imposed on the recruit.—The recruit and soldier hearts, how acted on by mechanical causes.—The heart, for example, compared with a pump.—Re-vaccination during recruit's drill increases the heart's action.—How squad drill, as a cause of disease, by suddenly altering the shape of the chest, interferes with the circulatory process.—Nervous and mental causes.—The balance of nerve-force at the heart may be upset by stretching the neck and chest.—Evidences of the direct action of the state of the brain on the heart (Claude Bernard, Darwin, etc.)—The disturbing effects of drill, and suppression of feelings, cause this direct action.—First indications of the recruit's heart being unduly acted on.—Sudden changes of life disturb the mental faculties and cause disease.—Examples of mechanical effects and mental effects.—References to foregoing influences.—Parke's experiments on the effects of carrying the knapsack.—Remarks on the use of dumb-bells, and the nature of parade work.

HERE then, having considered, as it were, the first stage of man, the other two may be treated of as the recruit's and the soldier's. But it will be convenient not to divide them too distinctly, for practically they glide one into the other. We shall see presently that the bearing of the drilled soldier differs so from that of the raw recruit that during the transition stage the heart must be displaced.

Now it may be well, in the first place, just to note and thus call to mind, what takes place in that period, during those early days in which defects of the circulatory system are created and disease so remarkably and extensively developed. (1.) The recruit having enlisted, is as a rule washed before medical inspection. This is his first sanitary lesson; for all previous arrangements of the parochial or municipal authorities were looked upon in much the same light as the uninitiated always do on direct and indirect taxation—they hear of one, but they feel the other; but the simple fact of being ordered may excite the imagination or produce strange feelings in one who has inherited independence and just forfeited it perhaps to get away from the restraint of his parents. (2.) When found physically "fit," sworn in, and brought under dicipline, he is handed over to the drill instructor, and also taught his first lessons in subordination. (3.) In the meantime, he is vaccinated, and dieted on a scale generally better than what he has been accustomed to, probably previously being out of employment or dissipating. (4.) When clothed, accoutred, served out with a kit, numbered, sufficiently instructed, with his chest expanded and its shape altered, he joins the ranks as a soldier, and then becomes liable to those incidental conditions of his new career, perhaps among which we may consider tropical service, prison life, and war risks.

In proceeding to investigate this subject further, it seems advisable to consider it, as regards the individuals acted on, from both a mechanical and a mental or vital point of view. Now looking at the heart in the light of a purely mechanical instrument, divested of all vital properties and barrack-room associations of beer and tobacco—take for instance a pump fitted up and working smoothly for years in a certain position, in a space suitable for its accommodation—removal from that position and any alteration in the space assigned to it, will most probably throw it out of gear, and if at the same time it is obliged to force a somewhat denser fluid, under higher pressure than usual, through tubings which have their position and curvings altered, it may not be found equal to the test. Now this is the test to which the heart of every recruit is subjected. Before going further there are two points here which may require explanation —"a denser fluid under higher pressure." It is probable the generality of recruits receive more blood-forming food than pre-·viously accustomed to, and when the fluid is more dense than usual, there is more strain thrown on the heart ; but the same cause will strengthen the heart, yet these things may affect it. The second point has reference to constitutional irritation set up by re-vaccination stimulating the heart's action. That vaccination permanently quickens the pulse has been denied, and the idea abandoned; but Dr. Seaton, in *Reynolds*, remarks :—" Severe constitutional symptoms are out of all proportion more frequent in re-vaccination than in primary vaccination."

Every recruit is re-vaccinated while going through his setting-up drill; few become sufficiently ill to be admitted to hospital or even excused drill; still all are more or less constitutionally affected, or rendered feverish.

As regards the drill instructor, by suddenly and almost violently altering the shape of the chest, the heart is thrown out of gear; by stretching the neck, and altering the curvings of the spine, and straightening the dorsal region, the chest is carried forwards and upwards, the muscles of the back are contracted, while the abdominal are strained; and these latter, by reason of their attachments, drag down and fix the inferior ribs, and sternum, and tend to pull the side walls of the chest into a narrower compass, and drag down the attachments of the diaphragm —that powerful respiratory muscle. The whole arrangement seems to have more a tendency to lengthen and perhaps narrow the lower portion of the chest than expand it; to compress the liver, which is brought below the ribs, not so much on account of the weight of the gland losing some of the pressure of the abdominal viscera, as because of the diaphragm being brought lower, on account of its attachments to the ribs; the crura are also put on the stretch, for in the new position the curve of the lumbar vertebræ is increased and carried forward under the centre of gravity. As the pericardium, where the heart resides, is attached to the diaphragm, it is also brought lower down, or more suspended from its direct attachments, it is undoubtedly interfered with, and the aorta is stretched and has its curvings altered.

It is the lower portion of the chest that is principally affected, from about the region of the heart downwards; but the upper portion of the frame-work appears altered in shape, for the blade bones and arms are thrown back, and the neck stretched and carried back, and because of the dorsal curve being somewhat straightened, the chest is tilted forwards and upwards; but from the fixings and position of the upper ribs, necessary to give attachment to the pectoral muscles, the shape of this portion of the cavity of the thorax cannot be at all easily altered, and it is able to resist, even in youth, the efforts of the drill instructor. But in more hardened individuals of the recruit's class, where bone and muscles are developed, I expect it is a great source of annoyance to get a proper arrangement of these parts, especially if the clavicles are short and curved. In women the lower part of the thorax is not much called into play in the respiratory process peculiar to the sex, as by nature they are unsuited for severe manual labour, and abdominal or costo-inferior respiration would be impeded during gestation, or the gravid womb disturbed. In the upper classes of society especially, apparently from the pectoral muscles and those of the upper extremities not being much developed, or requiring firm support, the upper portion of the chest is very little fixed; thus they bear pressure about the lower ribs wonderfully. While with the opposite sex it is the upper portion resists pressure with least inconvenience. Thus it is, an amount of restriction about the waist sufficient to extinguish a recruit, a lady can bear with ease. I wonder if women accustomed to manual labour suffer from impeded respiration to any marked degree during gestation.

How far the heart is displaced by suddenly altering the shape of the chest, cannot be ascertained, it will so vary in different individuals. No given rules in connection with bony landmarks or the nipple can be of use; it will be principally in regard to its relation with the diaphragm and sternum, downwards, with its apex inclined towards the centre. This changes the direction of the heart's axes, and brings it more in line with the ascending portion of the aorta, which will be stretched and straightened, so that the blood may possibly strike more directly against the great sinus, the most usual site for aneurisms.

Thus, having observed the heart from a mechanical point, as a machine working smoothly for years in a certain position, one ought not to be surprised if it gets out of order when the experiment is tried of making it carry on its work in a new position. Now I think we have shown that the heart of the recruit is obliged to work in a new position, for during the first few months of a soldier's career every legitimate means, short of actual violence, is taken to rip up old adhesions and remodel the hereditary shape of the man, and above all, to alter the shape of the thorax by a so-called expansion, thus interfering directly with his heart and lungs; and this is done so quickly in these days of modern improvements, by means of dumb-bells, clubs, and "extension movements," all combined into a system, directed to this one object, that the heart has not sufficient time to accommodate itself to the altered conditions against which it has to contend. It is this, even more than the degree of displacement, that interferes with its action, and this of itself, in very many cases, is sufficient to account for its equilibrium being destroyed, and the irritability of action it takes on in young men so soon after joining; and naturally, as one might expect, the younger and more pliable the individual, the more quickly and surely will he be thus affected.

Well, to consider the subject from another point of view, we must remember that the heart is not a purely mechanical instrument, but that it is intimately connected with organic and animal life, wonderfully endowed with irritability, and subject to be influenced by the emotions. Its irritability and vitality are due to nervous agency, and it may be worthy of notice that it receives its principal supply from nerves that arise in the neck, and they are liable to the same amount of pressure as the arteries in this region, and some of them to even more direct pressure; but what influence this may have on nerve-force, by interrupting it, or interfering with its currents, cannot be ascertained. I do not attach much importance to this altered position or stretching of the neck, or external pressure, for the heart seems very independent of its cervical supply as regards its irritability, yet Dr. Fothergill remarks: "Rhythmical irregularity is due to halting, hesitation, or partial arrest of the ventricular contraction, which may be brought about by a disturbance of the balance of power between the vagus and cardiac ganglia." Thus these causes may disturb the balance, and pressure at the root of the neck is more likely to induce an irritability of the heart through nervous agency, by disturbing the natural currents of nerve-force to be transmitted to the heart, than the same pressure is at all likely to do by interrupting the current of blood in the common carotid artery. Perhaps it would not be considered out of my province here to state that, as well as the vagus, which seems the motor-nerve, the heart is supplied from the three cervical ganglia of the sympathetic, the recurrent laryngial, and perhaps the phrenic.

Darwin, in his book on *Expression of the Emotions in Man and Animals*, 1872, writes : "The heart, which goes on uninter-ruptedly beating night and day in so wonderful a manner, is ex-tremely sensitive to external stimulants. The great physiologist Claude Bernard has shown how the least excitement of a sensi-tive nerve reacts on the heart, even when a nerve is touched so slightly that no pain can possibly be felt by the animal under ex-periment; hence, when the mind is strongly excited we might ex-pect that it would instantly affect in a direct manner the heart, and this is universally acknowledged and felt to be the case. Claude Bernard, also, repeatedly insists, and this deserves special notice, that when the heart is affected it reacts on the brain, and the state of the brain again reacts through the pneumogastric on the heart, so that under any excitement there will be much mutual action and reaction between these the most important organs of the body."

During recruits' drill, owing to the disturbed state of the men-tal faculties, individuals being perplexed, annoyed, or otherwise agitated, a large amount of nerve-force is generated by the vesicu-lar neurine of the cerebrum, in the ordinary course of events to be transmitted to the muscles, and this force, under the natural or ordinary conditions of life, where man is a free agent and free from the restraint of discipline, would be expended in muscular efforts—by gesticulations, walking up and down, or by letting those who gave rise to such feelings partake of his mind. But no such safety-valve is open to the soldier. On parade all such voluntary expressions of the emotions, by word or gesture, are strictly forbidden, and we shall see that it is a fact, that under these conditions they do manifest themselves in the first instance in those muscular efforts which are *involuntary and most habitual in their action*. Here, then, as the heart's action is involuntary, and the most constantly worked organ in the body, it of course will be the first and mostly affected if any causes should give rise to mental disturbance in the soldier. Now to verify this statement, and to apply it further to the service. Darwin again remarks: " Why the irritation of a nerve-cell should generate or liberate nerve-force is unknown, but that this is the case seems to be the conclusion arrived at by all the greatest physiologists, such as Müller, Virchow, Bernard, etc., and Mr. Herbert Spencer remarks: 'It may be received as an unquestionable truth that at any moment the existing quantity of liberated nerve-force which in an inscrutable way produces in us the state we call feeling, *must* expend itself in some direction, *must* generate an equivalent manifestation of force somewhere, so that when the cerebro-spinal system is highly excited, and nerve-force liberated in excess, it may be expended in intense sensations, active thought, violent movements, or increased activity of glands.' Mr. Spencer further maintains that an overflow of nerve-force undirected by any motion, will manifestly take the most habitual routes, and if these do not suffice, will next overflow in the less habitual ones."

Thus it may be seen that the heart will be first affected and in a most direct manner, and next the respiratory organs, which are but partially under control of the will. This granted, and even independent of parade work and incidental causes, let us see how an excess of nerve-force is generated in the recruit. Müller says: "Any sudden change of condition of whatever kind sets the nerve principle in action." Now the recruit's condition is certainly undergoing a sudden change, a change unknown in civil life; he is just embarking in a new sphere of life, with all it strange surroundings and regulations, which lead to mental disturbance, anxieties for the future, and a certain amount of nervous strain, with suppressed feelings. It is unnecessary to be acquainted with the service to understand the baneful effects these conditions of life will tend to exercise on the heart. While on parade, if we observe a recruit or soldier sigh, through pent up feelings, bewilderment, anxiety to ask questions, worry or suppressed rage, disturbance of the sensorium is taking place —nerve-force, the dynamic principle of vesicular neurine, is being liberated in excess, and after flying to the heart, we merely see the manifestation of its overflowing in the next most habitual route, which is but partially under control of the individual; or again, if you observe a tear in the eye, through an involuntary over-secretion of the lachrymal gland, a quiver in the nostril or lip, or, what is common enough, perspiring without any great muscular effort, or a trembling of the muscles, you may rely on it that the seeds of an uncontrollably irritable heart are possibly being laid in the whole squad. It is unnecessary here to dwell further on these nervous influences; the whole bearing of the case becomes palpable after a few moments' reflection, and it can easily be understood how directly they lead to functional derangement of the type met with in the service.

By regulation it is laid down how carefully the recruit is to be dealt with : "The instructors must be clear, firm, and concise in giving their directions; they must allow for the different capacities of the recruits, and be patient when endeavour and good-will are apparent; recruits should fully comprehend one part of their drill before they proceed to another, etc." Yet practically, and to a degree necessarily, while being taught there is a good deal of irritation one way or another. Men are required in the ranks, and must be put forward; and with respect to the firmness of drill-sergeants while either admonishing or directing a squad, numerous amusing illustrations may be found in *Punch*, and they have a very practical bearing on this subject.

Here then are the mechanical causes, and the nervous or mental causes, that give rise to heart disease in the army—that irritable functional derangement peculiar to the soldier, a palpitation often accompanied by irregularity in the rhythm of its action; and while this of itself is the cause of most heart disease recorded, it is also the source of most other affections of the circulatory system. I believe it is the displacement of the mechanical arrangements of the circulatory apparatus, so that the heart is obliged to perform its functions in a constrained or abnormal position, without sufficient time to accommodate itself to the altered conditions, that is the chief cause of "palpitation." The position of attention is typical of the position to be adopted on all duties, only departed from by the necessity for locomotion, and it is also typical of the abnormal position which throws the mechanism of the circulation out of order. It is not the over-work of the individual, the physical labour of recruits' drill or running drill, calling for increased heart's action to supply blood to the tissues, or the wearing of accoutrements, as generally stated, that disturbs the equilibrium of the circulation in the first instance ; but its having been disturbed renders men incapable of performing such active duties. These can merely be looked upon as accessory or secondary causes ; drill and discipline, the primary. When originally induced by setting-up drill, pal-pitation recurs whenever the man has to adopt for any little time the perfectly erect position, which is the exciting cause ; con-sequently standing at attention on parade for those who are thus affected—not through nervous agency—is the most certain way of producing its recurrence. I have recently seen a capital example of this sort in a marine on board the flag-ship at Port Royal, Jamaica. The man used to work hard and willingly, but to stand on deck at attention even for a few moments, unarmed and unaccoutred, he could not. Cases of this description are of daily occurrence in the service. But taken altogether, this pal-pitation of heart is brought about by a struggle to carry on its own allotted functions under displacement and suppressed men-tal emotions in those subjected to military dicipline, with all the worry and anxiety attendant thereon. It is this, by giving a per-petual unhealthy strain to the nervous centres, reacts on the heart and disturbs its action, by probably disturbing the balance of power concentrated in the cardiac ganglia. The struggle is not to overcome obstruction, though this in a manner may affect it, but it is to carry on its own vital functions under altered conditions that constitutes the first fruits of disease. It is then the dynamic power of the heart that is at fault, directly being interfered with through internal causes, and alteration of its relations or connection with other organs in the chest, and not indirectly by external pressure obstructing the circulation, and it is also the dynamic power of nervous agency being interrupted or otherwise interfered with in the free flow of its natural currents, that throws its full power directly on the heart.

At Barbadoes, only the other day, while a detachment of the 2nd West Indian Regiment were quietly awaiting the arrival of the general to inspect them at shelter trench drill, two of the men fell down with fluttering of the heart and giddiness—the usual thing. For some days previously they were practising this drill, all apparently in good health. Now what made these men fall out? what knocked these negroes down? not fatigue or tight clothing? No; they were anxious if possible to excel the 35th Regiment, who were inspected at the same work a few days previously.

I shall now refer to one of the late Dr. Parkes's experiments, which seems rather to substantiate my views, and the more readily, because it may be construed into an argument against my opinions. At page 576 he writes: "The production of heart disease ought not to be attributed solely to the knapsack, as is sometimes done; the knapsack is only one agent; the cross-belt was probably worse, and the tight clothes add their influence; but even with the knapsack alone the effects on the pulse is considerable, and one or two of my experiments may be given in illustration. Thus, four strong soldiers carried the old regulation knapsack, service kit, great coat, and canteen, but no pouch and no waist-belt (except in one man). The pulse (standing) before marching was on an average 88; after 35 minutes it had risen on an average to 105; after doubling 500 yards, to 139, and in one of the men was 164, irregular and unequal; after the double they were all unfit for further exertion. In another series, the average pulse of four men with knapsack only was 98 (standing); after one hour's march, 112; after doubling 500 yards, 141. If the pouch and ammunition is added, the effect is still greater." Of course, naturally the effect would be greater, but I think it is the position the knapsack makes the men assume, as if a back-board were worn, by drawing the scapulæ together, straightening the back, and tilting forwards the chest, and not altogether physical labour or the pressure of straps, that was the cause of all this acceleration of the circulation ; for in the first instance four men carried a great deal of weight, and after doubling 500 yards, the pulse rose from an average of 88 to 139, while in the next trial the knapsack *only* was carried, and after doubling 500 yards the pulse went from 98 up to 141. This argues more for unfavourable position than exertion or external pressure of belts, as simply carrying the pack raised the pulse 43 beats, and when carrying all their belongings 51 beats, a difference of 7, which is certainly not above what one might expect, all things being equal, from the increased effort of carrying weights even under favourable conditions. But there is a limit to the rapidity of the heart's action, so the last lot were handicapped by starting at 98, for the lower they commenced the better chance of a high average on the difference; again, there was no time taken. I believe it has been proved by experiments that the Prussian pack was easier carried than ours, a circumstance more probably due to its fitting round the man's back than to the centre of gravity being lower down, for with them the pack was made to fit the shape of a man's back, and not the man fitted to the pack. We issued out flat packs, and the drill-sergeant was at his wit's end to make round backs flat to fit them; but be this as it may, they are a thing of the past; and since the improvements of the Committee of 1864 have been tried for years, we see the amount of disease has not been reduced. Thus the cause must be sought for *de novo*, and I am convinced that we must look to the drill instruction in the barrack yard, in conducting the regulation *extension movements in order to open the chest* with his dumb-bells, back-boards, clubs, and other modern appliances for expanding and altering its shape, and thus interfering directly with the heart's action, and also to the manner in which discipline is enforced, and internal economy conducted, and not to the "Royal Factory at Pimlico," to account for the enormous amount of disease, human suffering, and loss to the state.

Now by reference to the regulations laid down for dumb-bell exercise, we shall see that there are a combination of influences or conjoined modern improvements at work which must affect the chest quicker than formerly, when the system was not so perfect, and thus how little time is left to the heart and lungs, "which ought to be educated, so to speak," to accommodate themselves to the new conditions of the frame. At page 6 we read : "The position and movements are of the highest order, and are directly and powerfully conducive to erecture of carriage and freedom of limb, and for these reasons they may be advantageously added to the setting-up and position drill of the recruit." If I am correct in my views, there is nothing in the whole physical training of our young soldiers costs the state so dearly as dumb-bells. I should much like to see them discontinued. The shock from dead metal at arms' length in endeavouring to expand the chest is undoubtedly very *direct and powerful*, far different from the swing of clubs, or unarmed hands. Dumb-bells are too powerful instruments to be left under control of drill-sergeants. I believe even when judiciously used by young men of their own free will going in for training, they tend towards heart derangement. In this latter class, from over-training or from fatigues following prolonged or over-exertion, excitement, and nervous tension, they often develop certain derangements of the heart.

While awaiting parade the mental faculties are generally disturbed by a foreboding anxiety, slight it may be, but still existing; for it is a very rare thing to have a parade without some one going wrong, being "dropped on," or found fault with. In marching the soldier must maintain the head and body at the position of "attention." This abnormal position gives a considerable muscular strain, which makes parade-work for infantry very tiresome, more especially when it is not enlivened by any novelty in the battalion movements, or variety in the manœuvres, while the position of the man is also unfavourable for the action of some respiratory muscles, and these are the things which principally rob parade work of what it otherwise might be, a healthy out-door exercise. Again, taking authorised regulations, in the introduction to the *Gymnastic Exercise* we read : " All exercises of mere position or posture have been avoided, for in no way do they furnish adequate exercise to the healthy adult, the recognised normal condition of the soldier.   They are in fact to his great requirements and capacity for physical exertion, but a tantalisation. Moreover they are quite incompetent to maintain in their practice the pleasure and interest which are essential to the beneficial result of all exercise."

Well, it may be said, if setting-up drill, parades, guard-mounting, internal economy, discipline, etc., were the cause of preponderance of functional derangements and heart affections generally in the army, the best set-up and smartest regiments would be expected to suffer most.   Not necessarily, for in the first instance smart regiments have more selection of recruits, and the commanding officer rejects those whom he considers of a bad type; and in the event of these men afterwards enlisting in other corps, they may get over-drilled while endeavouring to make anything like respectable-looking soldiers of them.   Besides getting a better class of recruits, favourite corps can spend more time in passing recruits through their drill, as they get a more abundant supply of the raw material, consequently the chest will have its shape altered or judiciously expanded, and not opened like an oyster by the drill instructor.   Naturally well set-up recruits will not be subjected to this, and if intelligent, they will not be so liable to be perplexed and worried.   Again, a great deal depends on the instructor, for no matter how zealous a man may be in the discharge of his duty, if he gives rise to such feelings as are likely to react on the heart, it is probable he will not turn out his recruits as smart and well set-up as those under the guidance of a more even-tempered and common-sense man.   If this be granted, without going further, we may say that men of the best set-up regiments are not necessarily the most subject to heart affections.   The Guards are extremely well set-up, and the men are taller than the generality of our troops; yet they show a smaller percentage of these affections than other arms of the service. Their recruits are selected from a more intelligent and better class, and their instructors are the best in the army; yet as they are not subjected to the injurious and depressing effects of foreign service, which seems one great cause of developing these affections, they cannot be admitted as a case in point.

Having thus far observed the subject from an infantry point of view, and those that are well set up, let us pass on to a branch of the service where we find men without any pretensions to be well set-up; for the disability under consideration pervades the entire army, and is not confined to men who wear packs and belts. Instance drivers in the Royal Horse Artillery; they are not well set-up, but they get driving and riding-drill sufficient to arouse evil passions, the baneful effects of which react on the heart in an equivalent degree to what others are subjected to on foot-parade; besides, there is no class of men in the service so forced through their setting-up drill, to get them into stables to clean their horses, all batteries being under-manned. These men wear no accoutrements; their work is undoubtedly hard, and being principally about harness-rooms and stables, is for the most part performed in shirt-sleeves, their full-dress jackets are not tight, there is no violent over-straining, they get very little night duty on stable pickets; guard-mounting is done by the gunners. If dress and accoutrements were the cause of so much disease, these men ought to be almost exempt from it; but such is not the case. Now observe the police force; their setting-up drill is never overdone, and if some at first have their circulatory system over-taxed through altered position, they get years of slow work and hours of relaxation to recover; consequently, as proved by statistics, heart affections among them are far less prevalent than in the army. They are subjected to the pressure of uniform and the effects of night watching, which has been by some supposed to affect the heart; but these men have a differently applied system of discipline, and from the nature of their duties and whole tenure of life, no comparison can be drawn between the police force, or fire brigade, and regular troops. Much the same may be said of the volunteers, and they, like school-boys, drill for their own amusement. In the latter the tissues are very soft and elastic, and they may be altered in shape, or prevented assuming certain positions, as the bones have not ossified into their hereditary formation; but the recruit has all old adhesions, mental and bodily, broken up, and his drill is for the most part carried on under depressed feeling, anxieties for the future, or other disturbances of the mental faculties. Mr. Myers, in his essay, comparing the army with the navy, says: "The navy, it might naturally be assumed, would show a greater death-rate from this cause than the army, owing to the abnormal strains frequently imposed on the sailor's heart by the extreme and sudden violent exertions which are incidental to his work." He then draws comparisons from six years' observations, which show the navy mortality at ·66, and invaliding 3·44 per 1,000, while during the same period the army mortality was ·9 and the invaliding 5·26 per 1,000. Here is a point worthy of attention, for doubtless, if such exertion were the cause in both services, the navy would show a higher percentage than the army; so there must be other causes at work in the latter service to supply such a high ratio of disease.

The navy is recruited from boys, and they are moulded into the requisite groove insensibly while pliable; they get a certain amount of drill, but are never over-strained at it. It is spread over a long period, and is looked upon much in the same light as a school-boy playing at soldiers, or being drilled at school. The thing is done gradually, and, as a rule, these boys do not feel restraint, for at their time of life they have never been free from it, while the recruit often rushes away from restraint only to subject himself to a more irksome discipline. Again, in the navy there is no sudden altering of the chest likely to give rise to the peculiar heart affection of the soldier. Discipline in the navy is very strict and exacting, but even if the ship is lying off shore, the men are not led into the same temptation as those

who have all the follies and amusements of the town at the
threshold of the barrack gate; thus they do not feel it so keenly.

Of later years heart disease seems to have increased in the
navy. Now this may be due to different causes acting with
various degrees of intensity: the increased amount of setting-
up drill, "small-arms drill," for adult seamen, and since flogging
is practically abolished,* there is a greater amount of imprison-
ment of latter years—prison on board is very different, both as
regards cell accommodation and diet scale, from what it is in the
army; further, owing to the introduction of steam, the staff of
stokers is greatly increased, and I am led to believe it is
among these men that heart disease is most prevalent, and apparently more on account of the variation of temperature to which
they are subjected while changing duties, than to hard work at
irregular periods, for, like all hands on board, they are kept at
regular work, although the ship may be lying at her moorings.
Although sailors are kept in constant training, so that like acro-
bats they seldom injure themselves, still of later years in the
different fleets, under intense excitement, when ships' crews are
competing with each other at such heavy drill as lowering
boats, etc., the men's feelings are pent up until the signal is
given from the flag-ship, then straining their vital energies to
the verge of destruction, they vie with each other. It would be
very difficult or impossible to prevent competition in these cases,
and if to these causes were added climate, conditions of service,
etc., they are sufficient to account both for any greater prevalence
of diseases of the circulatory system in the royal navy, as compared with what occurs in civil life, and also their increase in
that service of later years. The principal supposable causes of
this class of disease in the army certainly do not apply to the
navy.

In pursuing the subject further it would be well to refer to
some other races of men whom we employ as soldiers, in order, if

---

* Only fourteen seamen and marines were flogged in the course of the
year 1876, out of 35,000 afloat.—*Times.*

possible, to come at the whole bearings of the case, and get as broad a view of the subject as we can. I fear wrong conclusions have already been arrived at by observing the bearings of the case too much from a British infantry point of view; and thus the whole scope of the matter for investigation has not been dealt with.

The Sepoy, owing to his coming of an extremely well set-up race, seems not to be affected by his recruit's drill, and heart disease and aneurisms are not prevalent among these troops. We have before noted the idea that the erect bearing of Asiatics may be due to the custom, acting throughout generations, of carrying weights on the head; again, as some will have it, being "born soldiers," they of course go through their drill with pleasure; but how far this holds good I cannot say. It may be so, yet from the naturally lethargic bent of his mind and that of his native instructors being cast in the same mould, nerve-force is not generated sufficiently in the Sepoy recruit to arouse feelings of an irritative type, the suppression of which, if not expended in voluntary muscular efforts, as already pointed out, must react on the heart. What causes can be assigned for this difference, except race? Possibly climate; also diet and mode of living. As regards climate, he is equally affected with the white man by malaria, fevers, liver and splenic enlargements, and other tropical affections liable to cause that anæmic and dyspeptic condition which has been supposed to give rise to this peculiar affection of the heart. I do not think this great difference can be otherwise accounted for than by the original erect bearing of the individual and his natural disposition, and a differently applied system of discipline, which gives the greatest freedom of action while off duty. Taking two years' average in Bengal, the mortality of native troops from diseases of the circulatory system is only ·2C per 1,000, while in the same presidency, in 1871, an average year, the mortality for white troops was 1·6 per 1,000. I take these figures from Parkes. Now if we were to take the invaliding also into account, the case would be far worse against the British soldier; with respect to uniform, it could not effect the difference, for nothing tight is worn, and there are no packs carried in the East.

As our soldiers during the last few years are not sent to India so young as formerly, there may be a decrease, by-and-by, in the per-centage of heart affections from that portion of the army, as the men will show signs of the disability before their time comes for going abroad, and consequently they will be rejected as unfit; further, those who do go will have their recruits' drill completed previous to embarkation, and when they arrive in India, they will also have more stamina to resist the baneful effects of climate. The first hot season after arrival from home, it was customary to send young men to the hills, and it was supposed they developed disease while pursuing butterflies and other winged insects at these high altitudes, for the purpose of making collections of them. Although this in a measure may have developed or hastened disease, the mischief in most instances originated in the barrack square at the depôt; and hill stations, it appears from statistics, do not increase either heart affections or rheumatism.

From the East let us follow the subject to the West. Our West Indian regiments are by some supposed to be well set-up, and as they show a less amount of heart affections among them than the white troops serving in the same latitudes, it may be induced as an argument to show that recruits' drill is not a cause of this class of disability; but amongst these men we find the peculiar palpitation, though not to any great extent. Reference has before been made to two of these men falling out from nervous exhaustion of the heart, brought on through suppressed feelings under anxiety. The negro does not appear to me as what ought to be considered a well set-up man—nor can you make him so; for without reference to the lower extremities, which are rather remote from our subject, the circulation, there is either too much curve in the spine or too much muscle between the shoulders to obtain a flat-back; thus the profile of the chest is somewhat barrel-shaped. The shoulders in a well-bred negro are always carried high and square, which seems to take off from the neck. A good many half-breeds find their way into the ranks, but I am alluding to the unadulterated article. Again, owing to the position of the condyles of the occiput, the chin is protruded and the face turned upward when we want the desired effect. With the European soldier, while the neck is stretched and head carried high, the chin is not thrown forward, and can be carried with ease according to regulation. The African, although of a livelier disposition than his eastern congener, being cheery and happy under most circumstances and conditions of life, and of a different temperament, might still be considered as resembling him in the difficulty of disturbing, so to speak, the polarity of his nervous centres. While both nations, being either actually or practically subjected to slavery for generations, may have developed and inherited a disposition amenable to restraint, not so with the free-born Briton; his aversion to be interfered with in this way costs the state dearly.

White regiments serving in the West Indian command come direct from the United Kingdom and only remain three years on the station. They are therefore composed chiefly of young soldiers, at a time of service which gives so marked a prevalence to the class of disease under consideration. Consequently the idea started that those men stationed at Newcastle, Jamaica, where the white troops in that island are quartered, at an altitude of nearly 4,000 feet, was the cause of the comparative amount of these diseases, ought to be received with caution, judging from the age of the men and the statistics of hill stations in the Himalayas. The creole negro is not much addicted to drink, but if venereal was the cause of heart complaint and aneurism, we would find them exceedingly common in both sexes of this race, although the yaws and leprosy are said to be brought on by hereditary syphilis. I never heard the immunity of these people from yellow fever thus accounted for. The West Indian soldier still carries the old pack equipment, and here white troops seldom wear tunics.

4*

CHAPTER V.

Aneurisms, their cause of origin, etc.—Syphilis as a cause of origin.—Dr. Welch's opinion.—The amount of disease.—Inspector-General Lawson's and Dr. Maclean's evidence.—Death rate a mere trifle compared with the amount of disease.—The age of the men affected.—The remarkable absence of constitutional disease.—The fallacy of supposing syphilis to be a sufficient cause to account for the frequency of occurrence of aortic aneurisms.—Aneurisms in civil life, their chief cause of origin.— Evidence of the absence of disease of the vessel in many cases met with in the service.—Quotation from Myers.—Exercise.—Obstructions of dress and hypertrophy considered as a cause.—The situation in which aneurisms occur in civil and military life ; also in the different sexes.— The power of the heart considered as the chief cause of aortic aneurisms in civil life.—The supposition that so much disease can be due to syphilis, dress, exertion, etc., untenable.—The value of the " soldier's spot " as a proof that restrictions of the chest affect the heart of the soldier.—Quotations from Parkes.

IN a paper read by Surgeon-Major Welch before the Royal Medico-Chirurgical Society, on the 23rd November, 1875 (vide *Medical Times and Gazette*, 4th December, 1875)—" after pointing out that the causation of aneurisms [among soldiers] is not peculiar to climate, station, or occupation, nor connected with age, or any condition of the system brought about by length of service," he concluded from the medical history sheets of individuals, and evidences shown by *post mortem* examinations conducted at Netley, " that it becomes an incontrovertible deduction that the syphilitic virus must be regarded as a very potent cause in the development of the arterial lesion and its sequel, aneurism ;" and in a summary of the paper he states " that the chest constriction and temporary forced exertions to which soldiers are liable, act as adjuvants to the aortic disease in the production of aneurism, as fostering influences to the germs laid by syphilis, rheumatism, and alcoholism;" . . . "that in adopting preventative measures against aneurism, the attention must primarily be directed against the cause of aortic disease, notably the suppression of syphilis, and secondarily the conditions of dress, etc., which assist in its development. During the discussion which followed, Mr. Powell said "he thought army surgeons over-rated the connection between syphilis and aneurism; certainly disease of the heart itself was rather rare, and there was no instance of syphilitic heart disease in Mr. Welch's cases." Mr. Myers then expressed his opinion "that aortic aneurisms were greatly favoured if not entirely due to external constriction." Sir William Gull "believed syphilis might have something to do indirectly with the causation of aneurisms, but what proof had Mr. Welch that the patients were syphilitics save from these aneurisms."

Here, then, is the most recent discussion on this interesting subject with which I am acquainted; and although Mr Welch seemed very sanguine in the correctness of his views as to the causation of this disability, he does not appear to have carried conviction to his hearers. Therefore it may still be treated as an open question for controversy and further investigation, and worthy of the greatest attention, when we consider the vast importance of the subject both as regards the soldier and the state.

Now with respect to the amount of disease: Mr. Myers, writing in 1872, says :—

"It was but recently that an eminent physician expressed his opinion freely in military circles to the effect that he did not believe the heart disease of the army need be attributed to any exceptional causes, but to precisely the same as in civil life, the chief of which were rheumatism and Bright's disease. In consequence of this, all the invalids in Netley Hospital suffering from heart disease were one day collected together, and Dr. Parkes, at the request of Dr. Maclean, examined them. Of the total number, seventy, he found only two or three had any previous history of disease, rheumatic, renal, syphilitic, or otherwise, to account for the disease then existing; and he therefore expressed his unqualified opinion that the great bulk of these cases could only be attributed to causes which did not pertain to the civil population." . . . "In 1866 Inspector-General Lawson proved by statistics that deaths from aortic aneurism were eleven times more numerous in the army than in the male civil population (vide *Army Medical Report*, 1866);" but deaths from this disease give no real estimate of its relative extent in the two classes, for, like soldiers suffering from heart disease, many must leave the service thus affected and die ultimately from the same, their deaths being recorded in the civil statistics. "In illustration of this, Mr. Muscroft, of Pontefract, has informed me that, as Poor Law Medical Officer, he has had several cases of aneurism under his care, all of which were in discharged soldiers."

To verify still further this, I may add, Dr. Maclean (*Army Medical Report*, 1867) writes:—"Between the 10th March, 1863, and 10th March, 1869, 93 cases of aneurism of the aorta were admitted into the Royal Victoria Hospital. Of these, 7 died, and the remainder were discharged the service." Again, of another period he says :—"36 cases of aneurism of the aorta were under treatment; 18 were under 30 years of age, and 18 between 30 and 40. . . . The medical history sheets showed a rheumatic history in 5, and a distinctly syphilitic history in only 3 of the cases." There is no reliable information with which I am acquainted to justify the belief that the soldier is more afflicted with syphilis than the civilian. Certainly he is not to such an extent as that from this cause aortic aneurisms should occur, as they do, in all probability, say at least fifteen times more frequently among soldiers, for we see the deaths are a mere trifle compared with the prevalence of the disability. It would undoubtedly require a far greater amount of venereal than exists in the service to account for this difference. Further, the worst forms of syphilis are not met with in the army, undoubtedly not at home ; for the men affected are at the time of infection for the most part in good health, and living under hygienic conditions conducive to health, while they have great facilities for prompt and careful treatment of the primary disease. Moreover, should they drop into that cachectic state brought about by constitutional disease, and so liable to induce degeneration of tissues, they are relieved from all physical exertions likely to produce aneurism, and if unlikely to become again efficient, they are invalided and lost sight of.

Yet in the East, from whence most of Mr. Welch's cases came, through apparently a combination of malaria and syphilis, one meets with men saturated to a surprising degree. This mixture, if it be a mixture, pervades all tissues from the hair to the bones, and renders its victims utterly unsound. From the early age at which aneurism among soldiers occurs, and even from the circumstance that out of the numerous cases brought forward by Mr. Welch, in five only was the degeneration of the vessel tending to aneurism multiple, without signs of syphilitic heart affection or degeneration of other vessels being mentioned, one may be induced to suppose that probably they were not all of a syphilitic origin ; an abrasion of the aorta from any cause may take on a syphilitic action.

In military, as in civil life, I believe in the power of the heart will be found the originating causes of most aortic aneurisms. If syphilis were the cause of origin, why should it be limited to the spot in which aneurisms most frequently occur all the world over? The disease would be extensive, and in other vessels and tissues. Again, besides the remarkable prevalence of aneurisms in the army, the affection has a peculiarity, the same as observed of heart affections ; that is to say, its comparative frequency in the young. Even supposing syphilis were the cause of a good deal of disease, yet the older the soldier, the more likely would he be, leading a bachelor's life, to become constitutionally affected, and it is highly improbable that recruits who have been carefully examined for syphilis would be the very men after a few years' service to drop into a syphilitic state, and develop aneurisms so soon after joining ; for it is within the first three years' service that this disability is so strikingly prevalent among men of from 19 to 25 years of age ; while from the experience of Sir A. Cooper, it occurs most frequently in civil life from 30 up to 50. The cause of its occurrence and limitation between these latter years, that is during middle life, is well explained by the supposition that the heart retains its power of execution, and the mind its youthful vigour, at a time the arteries are losing their wonted resiliency—not through any abnormal defects; for aneurisms, according to the above authority, are exceedingly rare after 50, at a time the tissues are most prone to degeneration; *but then the heart has lost its power.* Thus in civil life we must look upon the heart as the primary cause in the majority of cases, and not constitutional infirmity brought on by gout, rheumatism, or syphilis. Furthermore, judging from the comparative absence of mitral valve disease in the army (an affection more frequently due to constitutional disease than a similar affection of the aortic valves), and the respective ages of the two classes we have been comparing, one might infer that constitutional diseases collectively are not as frequent a cause of diseases of the circulatory system in the army as in the male civil population; and as regards constitutional syphilis individually, from the circumstance of the number of aneurisms not being reduced since the inauguration of the "Contagious Diseases Act," which undoubtedly reduced the primary affection very much, and taking the whole bearings of the case into consideration, one might conclude that syphilis cannot be the cause, and is insufficient to account for the frequency of occurrence of aortic aneurisms. Syphilis, as Sir William Gull remarked, "has only something to do indirectly with the causation," that is, taken in a broad sense, for in some instances it may be the primary affection.

In that admirable publication, *Cyclopædia of the Practice of Medicine,* edited by Dr. H. Von Ziemssen, vol. iii., page 217, we read :—"Atheroma of the arteries, has, however, in many respects, so much similarity to the new growths due to syphilis, that it seems to be allowable to suppose a connection between these changes and that disease. It has been attempted, at various times, by Morgagni, Wilks, and others, to establish a connection between the formation of aneurism of the aorta, or of other arteries and syphilis, and this seems to be quite proper, in so far as this disease is the cause of atheromatous or other degeneration of the arterial walls." . . . "Amyloid degeneration of the blood-vessels may also be mentioned as a change which takes place in some way as yet unknown, in consequence of syphilis ; it is often first recognized in the vascular coats, and, as a rule, begins in the smaller vessels."

In the *Blue Book* for 1867, page 316, Surgeon Hyde, commenting on a case of aneurism that occurred in a man of the 2nd Dragoon Guards, says, "*The absence of atheroma* in the aortic coats deserves notice, and it will probably be evolved as these cases are more observed, that numerous instances of aortic aneurism in the army are unconnected with any special pre-existing structural degeneration of the arterial coats." This has been also observed by others, and is well worthy of note.

What other causes have been assigned for this great excess of aneurisms, if not of a constitutional nature, are due to the effects of climate, etc. Having already drawn attention to the probable connection that exists between this affection and palpitation, perhaps it would be well in the first instance to consider other supposable causes. Mr. Myers, in his essay, thus enlarges somewhat on the opinions of Dr. Hunter, before quoted ; he evidently considers the aneurisms due to hypertrophy— the hypertrophy to mechanical obstruction of the circulatory process. He writes:—"Granting, then, that syphilis and excess of alcohol may account for a certain number of the aortic aneurisms of the army, I would assign the production of the majority to mechanical obstruction to the circulation in the soldier when he is undergoing exertion, caused by the general constriction of his neck and chest by faulty clothing and accoutrements." He continues :—"The heart, as I have already pointed out, to overcome its difficulties, becomes frequently hypertrophied ; but the aorta has not the same power. The blood, propelled with great force by the left ventricle, and checked in its onward flow, produces a great strain on the thoracic aorta, and by frequently dilating it beyond its normal limits, must ultimately so weaken, or even lacerate, the elastic fibres of the middle coat as to allow of the formation of an aneurism, or of a permanent dilatation in that part of the vessel where the shock is most felt—viz., the ascending and transverse portion of the arch."

I have before, at page 17, drawn attention to his views, where he says "he is inclined to think" hypertrophy exists, but not recognized, because the heart does not exceed the normal growth of the adult heart, but I may again say, why, if the disease exists to any extent, should it remain limited, and escape the notice of so many accurate observers? Even since he advanced these views, Mr. Welch, who has had every opportunity, and evidently paid the greatest attention to the subject, made no allusion to hypertrophy as a cause of aneurism in the service, and merely looked on external pressure as of quite secondary importance. I have already pointed out how inadequate the explanation of external pressure being the cause of origin of the excess of heart affections in the service is, and tried otherwise to account for the occurrence of disease; the symptoms of functional derangement are not those of hypertrophy. Of course, if the affection was of a secondary nature, brought on by an effort of nature to overcome obstruction in the course of the circulation, hypertrophy would be very common indeed; but there is the strongest evidence against the supposition that it is of at all frequent occurrence in the service. It is not "the soldier's disease."

I remember, at Meerut in India, a fine old soldier of the 98th Regiment—a well-known man in the regiment—being admitted with aortic aneurism. Previously he had been very little in hospital, but during the first few years of his service he suffered a good deal from palpitation, which gradually wore off. After death his heart was found considerably hypertrophied. Now in this case I believe the hypertrophy to be due to the obstruction caused by the aneurism, and the aneurism to be caused by the palpitation. That is in order—palpitation, aneurism, hypertrophy; the two latter frequently co-existing, but taking origin from the first. In the case in point, it was when the hypertrophy was fairly able to overcome the obstruction, and organic disease established, that the man had apparently no difficulty in performing his duties, and did not come to hospital until he was utterly done.

Aortic aneurisms, it appears, occur in the same situation in military, naval, and civil life ; and as the latter classes are not subjected to any undue external pressure, one would be inclined to look for some other cause to account for situation. Again, it appears they occur almost with a relative frequency in the same situation in all three classes. So far there is nothing to point to pressure impeding the circulation, or syphilis, as the exciting cause. These aneurisms occur at one particular spot—the great sinus of the aorta. That is a bulging at the upper part of its first stage towards its anterior and superior side, caused by the constant impulse of the blood against it. After the aorta, the origin of the cœliac-axis, and its bifurcation, the carotid at its division (this is above where pressure comes on the soldier's neck), the axillary, and the external iliacs at the groin ; and of external aneurisms the popliteals are the most common seats of its occurrence. In all classes, internal occur more frequently than external, for nature has not provided protected vessels with as thick coats as those exposed to outward injury. Thus, when subjected to unusual pressure from the blood, those internal and larger arteries, not having the strength or inherent power conferred by muscularity, of moderating or resisting such pressure, give way. I think it well, in passing, to direct attention to these well-known facts, as they all bear more or less on the case ; and also the evidences of what has been observed in the opposite sex, may with advantage be applied to a subject demanding the fullest investigation. As regards sex, without quoting authorities, it may be stated in round numbers that males suffer twenty times more frequently from aneurism than females, and for obvious reasons ; from the nature of their employment, habits of life, and alcohol and syphilis. This latter disease, with the exception of a certain class, is in the first instance confined to males. Guthrie also observes :—" The exertion in general is infinitely

greater in the man than in the woman; and I think this, combined with the freer use of ardent spirits, a much more likely
predisposing cause than either *syphilis* or mercury." And again—
" The force of the heart, however," says John Hunter, " has some
power in operating as a remote or first cause of aneurisms."
[Note from Chelius's *System of Surgery,* page 203.] I
think we may quite safely conclude, as previously mentioned in
connection with Sir A. Cooper's statements as to the age at
which aneurisms occur, the more so as future experience is cor-
roborative of their correctness, that *in civil life, the power of the
heart is the chief cause of aortic aneurism, the active agent in
their causation.* It may be said that the artery is at fault in
the first instance to allow the heart to injure it ; but when
much more at fault as age advances, we do not find aneurism of frequent occurrence, so it will not detract from the conclusion. Now, then, let us speculate on another cause for the
difference noticed between the sexes. Suppose Laennec's observations are correct, and the size of the heart does bear a relation
to that of the clenched fist, as women have comparatively
smaller hands than men, their hearts will not have relatively or
proportionately the same power of injuring the aorta. This
speculative idea may yet further be advanced when comparing
the British recruit with those of Continental powers. It has
been remarked by Dr. Crisp, " as interesting to observe, that
the above proportion does not hold good for all aneurisms,
for those of the carotids are as frequent in women as in men,
and other aneurisms thirteen or nineteen (differently stated)
times more numerous in men." Even allowing for errors in
diagnoses, from the frequency of tumours about the neck, and
enlargements of the thyroid body in females, it is remarkable
that these cases occur so often. Moreover, as a rule women do
not wear clothes that cause any restrictions about the neck,
while soldiers, who are supposed to have aneurism brought on
by pressure about the neck and armpits, do not show any
increase relatively in aneurisms of the carotids or axillary
arteries over sailors or civilians. Nor is there any evidence to

prove that axillary aneurisms are more frequent in the infantry than other arms of the service, although they are the only men who suffer any restriction about the axilla. Again, females, although they develop other diseases by external restrictions of the chest and waist, do not show any increase in abdominal aneurisms, although somewhat liable to that strange form known as dissecting aneurism ; and although tightly laced up, and subject to nervous and functional derangements, they do not suffer from the same irritability of heart as the soldier.

If external pressure was the exciting cause of aneurisms, or heart affections either, its continuance would increase disease, and the older the soldier the more likely would he be, living as he does under the same conditions, to be affected. And again, in India, where the assumed cause is removed, and where the natives do not suffer, there is no diminution of disease from that portion of the army, and it still retains its peculiarity of prevalence in the young. This cannot be accounted for by acclimatization, as all other diseases increase with age, both at home and abroad. If violent straining or over-exertion was the chief cause, we should expect to have more aneurisms in the royal navy than the army; but such is not the case; in certain trades also they would be very prevalent. If mechanical obstruction by dress and accoutrements was the exciting cause, perpetuated by over-exertion at irregular intervals, we should expect to find fifty per cent. more disease in the infantry than the mounted branches, and at a time of life more approaching what is observed in civil life, at a time when the elasticity of the artery was becoming impaired by age, or may-hap constitutional disease affecting the vessel, because on field-days infantry are frequently called on to run about smartly, carrying accoutrements and ammunition, while the others, being mounted, are not subjected to a similar strain, and are accustomed to regular work about stables, forage barns, etc.; thus one might infer that the fault cannot be in the vessel, except perchance in a small proportion of cases.

I shall now refer to an anatomical or pathological appearance

of extremely common occurrence on the surface of the heart, to
which some importance has been attached since it has been
called "the soldier's spot." Mr. Myers says :—"To the soldier's
'spot,' to which special attention has been drawn by Drs.
Maclean and Aitken, I need not here refer further than to
record my recognition of it as one of our best proofs of the
frequent presence of an abnormal impediment to the free action
of his heart, and my belief that beyond this fact it has no important signification, nor in any way endangers life."

I have not seen what has been written by Drs. Maclean and
Aitken, or what the latter officer has written concerning the
"Growth of the Recruit"; but as regards the spot itself being
an evidence of the abnormal impediment to the free action of
the heart of the soldier, I am certain it is an error to suppose
that it is at all confined to the soldier.   There is on the
anterior surface of a great many hearts a whitish sort of thickening, a lymph-like deposit in the serous membrane or subserous tissue, quite as commonly met with on the heart of the
civilian as the soldier, and long known to students of anatomy as the "white spot of Baillie."   Dr. R. Harrison, in the
edition of his anatomy published in 1847, writes :—"On this
anterior surface a small white spot of variable size is often to
be seen, sometimes two or three, probably owing to the thickening of the serous or subserous tissue, the result of some slight
inflammatory action.   The late Dr. J. Hatch Power, my former
respected teacher, in his admirable description of the heart,
referring to the anterior surface of the right ventricle, writes :—
"In this latter situation Dr. Baillie has described a white,
opaque spot, like a thickening of the serous layer covering the
heart; it is sometimes not broader than a sixpence, at other
times broader than a crown piece; *it is so very common* that it
can hardly be considered as a disease."   After the evidences of
these anatomists, who derived their information from the hearts
of civilians, is it not manifestly incorrect to specially connect
this spot with the heart of the soldier, and bring it forward
as a "proof" of certain restrictions to his chest being a cause of

disease? Yet we must bear in mind that if this thickening is a deposit of lymph, brought on by some slight inflammatory action due to friction, it may be particularly well marked in those who were subject to palpitation. Parkes did not believe syphilis was the cause of so much heart disease as occurs in the service, and he wrote, as before quoted:—" *Whatever the cause* of the preponderance of diseases of the circulatory system in the army may be, it is probable they produce *both the cardiac and arterial disease.*" Thus he could not have considered these aneurisms to arise from syphilis ; and again he says, with respect to the effects of clothing:—"It appears to me, *if anything gives the tendency to heart affections,* then dress and accoutrements come in as *accessory causes,* and prevent all chance of cure."

CHAPTER VI.

Palpitation considered as a cause of aneurism in the army.—Accounting for their frequency of occurrence, age, situation, absence of disease, either constitutional or of the heart valves, aorta, or other vessels.—How palpitation causes aneurisms.—How apparently simple causes may induce aneurisms.—Difficulty of comparing other armies with ours.—Inference that absence from military duties, by reducing the amount of palpitation, affects the amount of aneurism.—Prolonged military service, judging from statistics, unnecessary for the production of aneurisms.—The relation which the size of the hand has to that of the heart, considered.—The recruit's class have probably large hearts.—The size of the heart, under the conditions in which the soldier is placed, probably induces aneurisms.

HAVING before pointed to the connection that exists between palpitation and organic disease of the heart, showing how the former as a cause of origin will account for the difference in age, pathological difference, and peculiarities observed between organic disease of the heart and valves in civil and military life, let us here try and connect the facts that palpitation, which is so exceedingly common among young soldiers, is the cause of the excessive amount of aneurisms that occur in these men. If the power of the heart is the chief cause of aneurisms in civil life, there is no reason why the same should not hold good for military life. Men are made of the same material, and we know that palpitation increases the heart's power. Why look further for the causation of the aortic affection ? Will not this simple fact account for all the differences noticed between aneurisms in civil and military life—the *frequency* of their occurrence, the *age* at which they occur in all arms of the service, in the cavalry and artillery, as well as the infantry ? It will also account for the *situation* in which they occur, and also their occurrence in those who have not suffered from *constitutional diseases, rheumatism, renal disease, or syphilis,* and when *the heart has been found in a normal condition,* and the *valves and aorta free from any form of disease or degeneration.* In pointing to this alliance of cause and effect between palpitation and aortic aneurism, it is worthy of note that when the former is not of frequent occurrence among men, neither does the latter affection exist to any marked degree; instance the police force, fire brigade, royal navy, and our East and West India regiments, as well as the civil classes of the community from which our soldier comes. If they originated from strains, as Surgeon Hyde supposed, why will they occur so notably in the elastic and pliable, and have their starting point exactly where the blood impinges on the vessel? As before stated, the increased action of the heart, by vigorously ejecting the blood (a small quantity it may be, and probably is), causes an abnormal and too frequent over-stretching of the aorta, and after wearing out the elasticity of the vessel, renders it flaccid, and thus having lost its most important attribute, aneurisms follow as a sequence to the primary affection. So far palpitation has a similar action to that of hypertrophy from obstruction, but the artery not being clogged with blood, as it would be in the latter case, the blood from the ventricle is squirted, without anything to blunt its force, directly against the side of the vessel. *This is why palpitation is so particularly destructive to the aorta.* In addition, the artery is placed at a disadvantage in the soldier, to resist the heart's influence, for, by altering the shape of the chest, and lengthening the thoracic cavity, the ascending aorta is somewhat stretched and straightened, for it is fixed above by the arteries that take origin from the transverse portion, and the heart being induced to descend from the position occupied previous to enlistment, close on the central tendon of the diaphragm, hangs, as it were, more out of the other end, and more towards the mesial line; so that, even if the heart were a passive organ, it would cause some undue stretching between itself and the origin of the arteria innominata, and reduce the natural curvings of the vessel, and this, together with the alteration in the direction of the axis of the heart, may cause the

5

blood to impinge more directly on the great sinus, or on some
part close by, not accustomed to resist such pressure. Yet the
heart is not a passive agent, and its force and frequency of action
are increased; thus each jet of blood tends to stretch and
straighten the vessel all the more. Either William or John
Hunter, I believe, considered the rush of blood, straightening
the aortic curvings, was the principal cause of the impulse of the
heart. Now the heart, which is the active agent, will be driven
in the direction of the axis of the jet of blood, that is downwards,
with a tendency towards the *left* side. These views as to the
direction in which the heart would be inclined from this cause,
have been questioned on high authority, but it must be remembered the artery is stretched as well as straightened, and it is
being stretched that straightens it in the direction from which
the blood came, owing to the diaphragm being brought down,
and the heart taking on increased action, an abnormal elongation
as well as expansion and straightening of the ascending aorta is
brought about. As a physical sign of palpitation, it may be just
as well to remark that the dulness never extends upwards; it is
always downwards.

It is the elastic longtitudinal fibres which form the basement
layer of the lining membrane, the "fenestrated coast of Henle,"
that are the most prone to undergo change of structure in the
aorta. Thus it can be easily understood how a tendency to
aneurism will be given by these conditions which cause an
unusual elongation of the vessel, and abrasions once commenced
by the wash of blood over the surface may stimulate or take on
various forms of disease. I merely mention these changes of
position to show that they probably have something to do with
the originating of aneurisms, by placing the artery at a disadvantage, although quite satisfied that the increased force of
the heart's action due to palpitation, where the blood is allowed
to strike home against the vessel, will in itself, all other causes
being equal, be sufficient to account for the excess of aneurisms
in the army. Other causes, and they are numerous, such for
instance as those of a constitutional or may be accidental nature,

as strains, acting as they do alike on both soldier and civilian, may be looked upon in their relation to palpitation as a cause of aneurism as of mere secondary importance; they, as it were, keep up the average between the two classes, but it is the excessive amount of palpitation that gives the excess of aneurisms in the army.

The simple act of being drawn up at attention on parade, on account of its causing a recurrence of derangement of the heart, is a fertile source of aneurism, and it occurs to me this is probably the most valid explanation of the prevalence of aneurisms among our young soldiers in India, where there are no restrictions of uniform and hours of relaxation, and not the same worry and anxiety attendant on their duties, which are carried on without undue exertion. Here it seems to be the continuation of the original exciting cause, namely, the abnormally erect position that provokes the heart's action, the active agent. Thus the recruit may leave his tunic and pack at home, but the latent derangement of his heart, excited during a few weeks' drill in the barrack square, he will carry in his breast, and every time he is called to "attention" there is a tendency to develop and finally establish it as an acquired habit of the heart. When from any cause—malaria, insufficient food, mental depression, over-fatigue, poisonous influences, or prison life—the system is brought below par, that portion of the human machine which has lost its tone will be the first to show signs of derangement. It was under such conditions the disability described by Dr. Hartshorne was developed in those who went through the privations of the Potomac campaign. Their symptoms were exactly the same as occur in our men. The Americans, I expect, were hurriedly drilled under great excitement, and it is reasonable to suppose, placed under stringent rules to preserve discipline during war when they were conducted to the front. Here, in the first instance, the nervous centres were unduly strained; in itself this may lead to nervous exhaustion, but in addition these centres became subjected to those pernicious and poisonous influences which produced anæmia, at a time when the free flow of their natural currents was perverted and thrown on the heart. It was this gave rise to the nervous irritability of its action. The damage was done before the anæmia commenced, and when the anæmia was removed the heart symptoms still remained. A similar coincidence has been noticed in our service among men invalided from the East.

For many reasons it is not at all easy to draw comparisons between Continental armies and ours, as to the causation or extent of diseases of the circulatory system. Tho armies of France and Prussia, it appears, do not suffer as much as ours, although more than the civil populations from which they are recruited. I believe restrictions of discipline and the manner in which it is enforced, and the natural disposition of a people, will mark the difference far more than any difference in dress and accoutrements. Here it is worthy of note that "in the French army nearly one-sixth are always absent on leave."—*Parkes.* Again, a writer in *Blackwood* says, at the outbreak of the war in 1870, one-fourth of the regular army was on leave. Now, if such were the case with our army, those diseases produced *in and by* the service, would be greatly reduced, and most notably palpitation and its sequence, aneurism. In the absence of information as to what extent this functional derangement exists in other armies, I may say, wherever we find a comparative immunity from aneurisms, there is reason to suppose it does not prevail to any very remarkable extent. Eastern nations do not suffer much from these affections, perhaps in a great measure due to indolent habits, may be diet also; neither do our Sepoys suffer. When they finish their duties they have thorough relaxation, they are never confined to barracks during certain hours of the day, they make their own arrangements about food, they are not inspected during meals, they shift for themselves more, and have greater freedom in many ways. I cannot see that prolonged military service is at all necessary for the development of heart affections, although other diseases collectively in our troops show an increase with age, even in a more marked degree than among the civil population. Heart disease is peculiar in this respect. From some circumstance or other, diseases of the circulatory system are not as prevalent among the population of France as they are in England; now this must upset all calculations in comparing the armies of the respective nations.

But in pressing this matter a little further in another direction, it is again worthy of notice, the relation the size of the heart may bear towards that of the hand. As the statement came from one of great observation and authority, let us see in what way it may apply to our recruits. English writers considered Laennec under-rated the size of the heart, as of those from among whom he drew the comparison, the greater number died of phthisis ; yet be it more or less, this will not affect a relative connection between their sizes, and the conclusions arrived at by English authorities are for the most part derived from observations taken from our labouring classes. Now obviously a hand enlarged by manual labour will be associated with an increased size of the heart, developed indirectly as a necessary consequence, and as our recruits are drawn almost exclusively from the working classes, by nature of their employments they acquire or inherit, as well as certain forms and conditions of mind and body, large hands and hearts. Now is it not reasonable to suppose that other armies, drawn as they are from various classes of the community, would be found naturally better set-up, and with smaller hands. Large hearts and strong will naturally be most liable to injure the aorta, or, being worked in an altered position, to get out of order. Anyhow, it may be considered a consolation, slight though it be, that if the British soldier has more diseases of his circulatory system than others of his profession, it is in part owing to his largeness of heart. In indirect proof that physical exertion enlarges the heart, I take the following from Dr. Boyd's tables—Aitkin, page 516 :—

From 14 to 20 years of age :—

			lbs.	oz.		oz.
Males,	... Average weight of Body,	...	68	0	... Heart,	7·61
Females, ...	,,	,,	... 63	14	... ,,	8.46

From 20 to 30 years of age :—

			lbs.	oz.		oz.
Males,	... Average weight of Body,	...	92	14	... Heart,	10·96
Females, ...	,,	,,	... 86	13	... ,,	9.08

Now, supposing these figures to be correct, we see the tables are turned, and the male, presumably from the nature of his physical employments, outstrips the female in the growth and relative size of his heart, for while he gains 24lbs. 14oz. weight, his heart increases 3·35, while in the female, who increased 22lbs. 15oz , the size of her heart only increased by ·62 of an ounce ; and tables like these are usually compiled from observations in hospitals or anatomy halls, from those accustomed to employ- ments where physical exertions are required in the males. So instead of having small hearts, as Mr. Myers supposed, it is at least as reasonable to consider that our recruits have compara- tively large hearts. It has been observed that in addition to aneurisms being most frequent in middle life, we find in England that it is the middle-classes that are most liable to this affection. Is it not likely that these well-to-do people have but recently sprung from those who worked their hands constantly, and thus they inherit large hearts, and by reason of not working this organ regularly or proportionably in their generation, to what their forefathers were obliged to do, they only exercise it at irregular periods for their own amusements, and thus often unwittingly lead to their own destruction.   Now the fact is, to a certain de- gree we make middle-class men of our soldiers. If proved that a man with a large hand had also a large heart either acquired or inherited through cause and effect, or by a correlation of growth, it would be especially necessary for him to take regular exercise, and to avoid irregular or violent exercise with such a powerful machine.

I cannot better conclude this chapter than with the following remarks by Inspector-General Lawson, which will be found in

the Blue Book for 1866 :—"Many causes have been assigned for
the frequency of diseases of the heart and great vessels among
troops in South Africa, none of which appear sufficient when
examined into. Of these, great exertion during the Kaffir wars,
the excessive use of boër brandy, tobacco, and carrying the knapsack, have been most dwelt on ; but the diseases have been as
frequent among men who went to the colony subsequent to the
last war, as they were during its continuance, and they are not
more frequent among those who indulge in "Cape smoke," or
tobacco, very freely, than among others who use them sparingly.
Of late years, troops have always had their knapsacks carried on
a march in that country, yet the frequency of this class of diseases
is, if anything, on the increase. Some other cause, or combination of causes, must therefore be searched for to account for their
great frequency, which, as has been shown above, though most
prevalent on the Cape station, has caused a high ratio of mortality on many others." After referring to numerous cases of
aneurism, he says :—"The condition of the lining membrane of
the aorta has not been specially noticed in most of these cases ;
and, therefore, it is probable it presented nothing very unusual.
In one of them it was extensively pitted, as described by Roki-
tansky to follow the wasting of the patches of atheromatous degeneration; in one of those already mentioned it was quite free
from any trace of this degeneration, and there was no valvular
disease in the heart, showing that the origin of the aneurismal
sac is really not necessarily connected with either of these, though
they may be frequently found together in the same subject.
The immediate cause of aneurism, I conclude, from the facts mentioned in the former part of these remarks, to be phlegmonous in-
flammation of a limited portion of the coats of an artery, followed
by abscess, or simply infiltration, which so weakens their resistance, as to permit of dilatation, which either leads to early rup-
ture, or the gradual formation of a well-defined sac, as already
described. The cause of valvular disease of the heart, on the
contrary, seems connected with a rheumatic diathesis, and in
this country generally accompanies rheumatic fever, with well-

marked affection of the joints.   Such cases of highly developed
rheumatic fever are extremely rare among the troops in South
Africa, but muscular rheumatism, implicating the parietes of the
chest, is particularly common during the warm weather, and there
are few persons whose occupations require them to take active
exercise, who do not suffer from it more or less, and not unfre-
quently to a disagreeable extent.   There is a great tendency,
too, at that season to an excitable condition of the heart, which
may be brought on by moderate exertion, or slight chill, though
there may be no physical sign of either pericardial or endocardial
disease."

CHAPTER VII.

Remarks on a few arguments that may be deduced against the opinions advanced.—Medical history sheets.—The difference between hypertrophy and palpitation.—Some causes that give rise to palpitation.—Why typical cases from each cause are not very frequently met with.—Enquiry into facts, showing why it is so difficult to cure palpitation in the soldier.—The effects of habit on nervous currents.—Contrasting hypertrophy with palpitation shows why the latter affection is so particularly destructive to the aorta.—Probable causes why men adopt a certain position when they fall out of ranks, and find more relief in walking up and down than standing on parade.—Comparing the treatment of recruit and remount.

IT may be said, if aneurisms are caused by palpitation in those individuals in whom they occur, a previous entry for palpitation would appear in their medical history sheets. Now the testimony of these sheets is too imperfect to be considered as reliable evidence on this point. If correctly kept, there may be an admission shown for dyspepsia, debility, or in fact whatever the original affection may have been considered which gave rise to symptoms of palpitation. Secondly, an objection may be raised that if palpitation is brought on by weakness, fatigues, anæmia, etc., a symptom of exhaustion as it were, how can it be supposed to injure the aorta, and give rise to all this amount of aneurism. It has before been pointed out how it so acts, however, Dr. Fothergill, writing of hypertrophy, says :—" We now know that it is a compensatory growth : and consequently the more perfect the hypertrophy, the less does the patient or any one else know of it. So palpitation, which has been regarded as over-action, and treated accordingly, will soon be seen to be an evidence of the muscular power being taxed or wanting, and that is connected with the want of power, and not the excess of it."

Granting that both affections are due to weakness, so far it
must be accepted, they will have the same power of injuring the
aorta. Still it is the different causes of origin that marks the
affections ; one is a muscular growth, the other a manifestation
of nervous derangement. Hypertrophy is owing to weakness,
and the muscle growth grants compensatory power to overcome
the obstacle with which it would be otherwise unable to cope.

Palpitation due to weakness or nervous exhaustion is in the
same sense a compensatory power, in the dynamic nerve-force
concentrated in the heart, which is not controlled or kept within
bounds, but as there is no obstacle to overcome, and the heart
is equal to the task, there is no muscular development—its
action is excited through nervous agency, and its power and
frequency increased. As hypertrophy may be said to be due to
an effort of nature to supply blood to the system, so is palpitation owing to an effort of nature to rid the system of surplus
or misapplied nerve-force.

As nervous derangement or nervous exhaustion originates
from different sources, it is thus liable to be reproduced by
different causes. Exposing the individual to the exciting cause
is the most certain way of obtaining its recurrence. A body of
men exposed to the same conditions, unless they are so varied as
to catch the weak points of all, will not affect individuals in a
similar degree. If the cause of origin be the displacement of
the mechanical arrangements of the circulation, by interfering
with or displacing the heart, while altering the shape of the
chest during setting-up drill, without time for the heart to adapt
itself to the new position, by causing such a man to stand at
attention you adopt the most certain way of producing a recurrence of the affection. Here the muscular exertion or mental
anxiety is not great, but you place the man in the position that
first upset the equilibrium of the circulation, or interfered with
the balance of nerve-force concentrated at the heart. When
excessive smoking is the exciting cause, or vicious habits or
poisonous influences—malaria or alcohol—give the start, the
same will apply, and in these cases the palpitation frequently

comes on at night, when mind and body are at rest. The prolonged systole and irregularity in the rhythmical contraction, observed in some typical cases of this description, may be obliterated by those other conditions to which all soldiers are subjected. Again, over-exercise, or exertions leading to fatigue, will give rise to nervous exhaustion of the heart, manifested in an irritability of action easily reproduced by a recurrence of the exciting cause—namely, physical labour. Nervous excitement will have a similar effect, and produce the same phenomena, but the exciting cause here being of an essentially nervous character, generated at the sensorium, whenever there is any suppression of feelings, foreboding anxiety, or other condition producing mental disturbances which react on the heart, the original cause being again aroused, we are most certain of producing its recurrence, and finally establishing the disease.

Typical examples of these instances are of every-day occurrence, although for the most part the disability is due to or characterized by a combination of all acting on all. It is the nervous strain and conditions of life to which soldiers are subjected by reason of their employments and the system under which they live. Whatever the starting point is, it seems to be these conditions that modify these symptoms so easily excited, and marks the peculiarity of the functional derangement met with in the service.

Let us here enquire further into the facts of the case. The soldier, more especially the young soldier, is subjected to annoyances and anxieties unknown in civil life. These tend to set the nervous principle in action, and cause nerve-force to be liberated in excess of the immediate requirements of the individual, and this *must* be expended somewhere in muscular exertion, active thought, or increased secretion. We know the soldier is constantly obliged to check or suppress nervous currents, so far as to prevent voluntary muscular action, and thus allow of their being expended, as they would be expended in civil life; and it is an undeniable fact also that where such suppression of expressing the feelings or emotions takes place, nervous currents will be directed towards the heart, because it is the most habitually used channel for them to take, and there become expended in an increased muscular action of that organ, a circumstance over which the individual has no control. He has no means of preventing their taking their course, or of preventing his heart beating. Again, from Mr. Darwin's interesting book, before referred to, another point or fact may be brought to bear on this matter, that is to say, the heart of the young soldier will be affected in a direct manner through *habit*, acquired or inherited: for all exertions, voluntary or involuntary, tend to increased heart's action, and, by reason of this, nerve-force becomes accustomed to be expended in this direction ; and further, on the principle of association, "when there is any sensation or emotion, pain or rage, which has habitually led to muscular action, it will undoubtedly influence the flow of nerve-force to the heart, though there may not be at the time any muscular exertion." Now is it not more than probable that in men of the soldier class, even while standing on parade, if anything starts the nervous principle into action it will be especially liable to affect their hearts, on account of habit and association, these men having sprung from those accustomed to and being themselves accustomed to physical labour. And on this same principle, once nerve-force becomes habitually expended at the heart through the increased muscular exertion of that organ called palpitation, whenever the nerve principle is set in action it will undoubtedly flow in this direction, because it is the most commonly frequented route. It occurs to me that there is a very practical bearing in these facts, and from what has been said, it may be deduced that palpitation is the *uncontrollable habit* of the compensatory power granted to the muscles of the heart to expend the surplus nerve-force that results from the amount generated not being got rid of by voluntary action. Thus, palpitation once started as a defect, can be brought about, perpetuated, or confirmed by any cause that sets the nervous principle in action, and, when finally the habit is fully established, even when only sufficient is generated without excess, for the ordinary supply of the individual, it will cause palpitation. This explains why it is so extremely difficult to cure the nervous derangement of the heart met with in the service, and thus it is, when the disease is but even partially established, it is so very easily excited as to be scarcely worth while keeping the man on, where there are so many causes acting in conjunction with the original cause to perpetuate it, unless we could grant thorough relaxation from military duties so that the habit would be out-grown. With regard to the functional derangement of the young soldier's heart, Dr. Maclean thus writes (vide *Army Medical Report*, 1867) :—" Once fairly set up, I doubt if it is ever really cured. I have kept young men under observation for months under the most favourable conditions as regards rest, diet, and medicine, but, on causing them to resume their ordinary dress and accoutrements, or to walk quietly about the corridors of the hospital, distressing palpitation immediately returned, making further exertion impossible."

I would suggest that men with palpitation be passed into the reserves at once, and not kept with the colours until utterly broken down. I may be wrong, but it seems little more than expense sending men who have been under treatment a few times with this affection to India; even if they last until the novelty of the change wears off, as soon as they become anæmic, or knocked up from climate, the disease will be established. So constantly do the symptoms arise when men are reduced to a debilitated condition by malarial affections, that quinine was supposed to have somewhat to do with this cardiac derangement. It is probable some men subject to palpitation were sent to India under the belief that relaxation without restrictions to the chest in that country would restore the equilibrium of the heart's action. Here it occurs to me that the fact of the people who have suffered from ague, after removal from the locality that induced the disease, and being free for years from any symptoms of an intermittent character, if unduly exposed to cold or hardships, or in the event of becoming ill, their disability will assume an intermittent character, where there is no lesion with which we are acquainted, and an apparent absence of the original poisonous influences that gave the intermittent type.   May it not in these cases be owing to the *habit* acquired during the previous disease that causes the nervous centres to stamp other affections with an intermittent tendency?   It is only when the system is reduced the habit becomes apparent ; the poison has gone, but it left its impression ; does not this seem as likely to be the case in many instances, as that there are two poisons acting at the same time, the one showing itself after remaining latent for years?   I read somewhere of a man who after a few days' experiment of plunging into cold water at a certain hour, and wrapping up warmly immediately on returning from his bath, brought on a feeling of chill, followed by heat, at the same hour at which he was accustomed to bathe; in fact he produced a sort of non-malarious ague. That proved, so far as it goes, that external influences can cause an involuntary *habit* of the nervous centres.   May not poisonous influences which produce the same symptoms have a similar disposition, and become manifest in after years when the system gets below par, unless the habit in the meantime is thoroughly outgrown?

I have noted the circumstance that a heaving of the chest, a sigh, or tear may be looked upon as indications of the pent-up feelings that are surely reacting on the heart of the soldier. It is quite unnecessary to dwell on this point further, and it is evident, all things considered in connection with his career, that they will sufficiently account for the preponderance of the special affection of the circulatory system in the army, and also the pathological differences observed between the valvular and organic diseases in the soldier and civilian.   The small quantity of blood sent forward at each throb of this nervously-excited heart will account for many physical signs and symptoms recorded in true instances of this derangement, in both our army and that of the United States of America ; it shows why the heart in many instances has to beat inordinately quick on the least exertion, without any sign of an undue supply of blood to the tissues.   I expect, also, it will account for the dicrotism which

Myers considers characteristic of the sphygmographic tracing of the pulse in these cases. When the tone of the aorta is good, that is to say, its elasticity perfect, the dicrotism is perhaps least marked, for the vessel is able in a measure tor esist the pressure of the blood, and thus does not permit of its being shot so clear of the valves as to allow of space for recoil; for by clinging round the blood closely, and squeezing it back as well as onward quickly, there in no time left for the pulse-wave to assume a double form. It is when the vessel is getting the worst of it, and the increased work is telling on it, that the deepest marked tracings will be observed. Now as a cause of aneurism, is it not more than probable that the small quantity of blood forcibly ejected is allowed to strike home against the aorta in this condition, while in cases where the aorta is filled with undistributed fluid the shock is broken, and the vessel thus protected? Attention has been drawn to the circumstance that the artery is most probably placed at a disadvantage in the soldier to resist the power of the heart—the active agent in the causation of the majority of aneurisms in both civil and military life.

The position men generally assume when they fall out of the ranks, not from over-fatigue, is that which tends to restore the chest to its original shape. They sit on some low seat or sloping ground, bending and bringing the scapules forward, by placing the arms round or between the knee; thus pressing the abdominal viscera against the diaphragm, they tend to restore the heart to its original normal position. Every army surgeon must have seen instances of this. It is a mistake stretching out and lowering the head of a man who feels this position comfortable; if left to himself he will come round sooner. Mr. Myers, I think, mentions instances in which men kept waiting on parade under arms found relief in walking up and down for a short time in rear of the battalion, and he supposed they experienced relief by the exercise stimulating the heart's action to overcome the obstruction to the circulation caused by dress. It may be so; but may no it also be that these men by falling out could lounge a little, an thus let the heart approximate more towards its original position, while they felt additional relief by reason of the muscular exertion diverting the nervous currents from the heart?

Perhaps here it may be just as well to draw attention for a moment to the different courses of treatment adopted with the recruit and remounts, and observe the advantages of the system applied to the latter. Remounts are purchased as three and a-half or four year olds, and are not taken into regular work until five off. One year at least is spent over the breaking-in. They are quietly handled, given their paces, and taught to carry themselves according to regulation; but when the horse has naturally a badly-set-on head, there is considerable difficulty in the matter, and often his wind suffers during the process; but there is no attempt made at any time to alter the shape of the chest, and in this way interfere with the heart and lungs, and of course he is not subjected to the same nervous or mental strain in being taught. At the same time, among troop horses there is a considerable nervous anxiety, and they are well aware of those trumpet sounds which interest or affect them. When officers are busying about going round stables, or when there is any unusual bustle, you may observe a look or glance of suspicion almost I think peculiar to these animals—a sort of "what's-up-now" expression and restlessness. I do not consider any comparison can fairly be drawn between animals selected on account of certain points and trained for one special purpose, such as race-horses and greyhounds, and the mode of training or handling our recruits or remounts.

CHAPTER VIII.

Quotations from Parkes's *Hygiene.*—The effects of military service.—Sir R. Martin, Mr. Myers, and army medical reports.—Discipline, internal economy, routine duties, drunkenness, prison life, etc. affecting the heart by producing nervous exhaustion.—Service in India, its influence on heart affections.—Conclusion, pointing to some improvements that might be made in the physical comforts of the soldier.

THE late Dr. Parkes, that great benefactor of the soldier, in the introduction to his work on hygiene, which I gladly quote, although scarcely within the scope of this little book, as it may arouse further interest in the subject, after referring to the cupidity of house-owners, and the neglect of sanitation of dwellings among the civil community, says .—"Analyze also the effect of such selfishness and carelessness as I have referred to on the nation at large, and we shall find that the partial gain to the individual is far more than counterbalanced by the injury to the state, by the discontent, recklessness, and indifference produced in the persons who suffer, and which may have a disastrous national result. It is but too commonly forgotten that the whole nation is interested in the proper treatment of every one of its members, and in its own interest has a right to see that the relations between individuals are not such as in any way to injure the well-being of the community at large.

"In many cases, again, the employer of labour finds that, by proper sanitary care of his men, he reaps at once an advantage in better and more zealous work, in fewer interruptions from ill health, etc., so that' his apparent outlay is more than compensated.

"This is shown in the strongest light by the army. The state employs a large number of men, whom it places under its own social and sanitary conditions. It removes from them much of

6

the self-control with regard to hygienic rules which other men possess, and is therefore bound by every principle of honest and fair contract to see that these men are in no way injured by its system. But more than this : it is as much bound by its self-interest. It has been proved over and over again that nothing is so costly in all ways as disease, and that nothing is so remunerative as the outlay which augments health, and in doing so, augments the amount and value of the work done.

"It was the moral argument, as well as the financial one, which led Lord Herbert to devote his life to the task of doing justice to the soldier, of increasing the amount of his health, and moral and mental training, and in so doing, of augmenting, not only his happiness, but the value of his services to the country. And by the side of Lord Herbert in this work was one whose name will ever be dear to the country, and whose life, ever since that memorable winter at Scutari in 1855, has been given up entirely to the attempt to improve the condition of the soldier."

I abstract the following from his chapter on the "Effects of Military Service" :—The recruit having entered the ranks, begins his service at home, and is kept at his depôt for some time. He does not go to India until he has completed his twentieth year, although he may take other foreign service earlier. We should expect his life would be a healthy one ; it is a muscular and to a certain extent an open air life, yet without much exposure or excessive labour ; the food is good (although there might be some improvement), the lodging is now becoming excellent, and principles of sanitation of dwellings are carefully practised ; although the mode of clothing might be improved as regards pressure, still the material is good. "There is a freedom from the pecuniary anxiety which often presses so hardly on the civilian artisan, and in illness the soldier receives more immediate and greater care than is usual in the class from which he came. . . There are some counterbalancing conditions : among the duties of the soldier is some amount of night work. . . Commanding officers should be informed how seriously the guard and sentry duties, conducted as they are in full dress, tell on the men, if they are too frequent. . . The habits of the soldier are unfavourable to health; in the infantry especially, he has much spare time on his hands, and *ennui* presses on him. . . The establishment of trades especially, which would not only interest the soldier, but benefit him pecuniarily, is a matter of great importance. It has long been asked why our army should not do all its own work. Give the men the hope and opportunity of benefiting themselves, and *ennui* would no longer exist. . . Among the conditions of the soldier's life adverse to health, enforced celibacy must be reckoned." He continues :—"The last point which probably makes the soldier's life less healthy than it would otherwise be, is the depressing moral effect of severe and harassing discipline. In our army in former years it is impossible to doubt that discipline was not merely unnecessarily severe, but was absolutely savage. An enlightened public opinion has gradually altered this, and with good commanding officers the discipline of some regiments is probably nearly perfect; that is to say, regular, systematic, and unfailing, but from its very justice and regularity, and from its judiciousness, not felt as irksome to the men."

Although discipline, through an improved system, is more strict than formerly, it is not so rigidly enforced; matters have improved, yet the rules for the maintenance of all military systems seem too hard and fast; they are either in themselves too stringent, or the means taken for carrying them out too exacting to exercise a beneficial influence on health, though men may be well housed, clad, and fed. The recent alteration of the hour at which men are required to be in barracks for the night, is a great boon to the British soldier—a most salutary measure, as he will thus have a greater feeling of freedom. Hence there will be less anxiety about returning in time, and the crime of returning too late, with its consequent punishment, which means more or less injury physically and morally, will be diminished.

Where there is a good internal economy with the details of which the men are perfectly acquainted, nervous strain is relieved. Men ought to see clearly the object and the advantages that will accrue to themselves individually from carrying them out; barrack-rooms ought to be made more homely, and while men are taught a prompt and implicit obedience to orders, those who enter heartily into the spirit in which they are given ought to be granted immediate indulgence, as freely given as punishments for any dereliction of duty. Threatening or putting the law in force to oblige men to carry on their work is not a wholesome measure in either civil or military life, yet it is the one to which the soldier is too frequently treated. A judicious and common-sense method of conducting discipline and internal economy leads to contentment and happiness among men; if not itself invigorating, it relieves nervous tension, and *has far more to do with the health of regiments than is generally supposed.*

Formerly our army was not so enlightened or educated as in the present day. Men and manners have improved. The independence of the classes from which our recruits are derived did not then exist. Now they feel in their own persons, or reason by analogy from their knowledge of things in general, that they have forfeited, like Esau of old, although not in so high a sense, their birthright of independence, and parted with some civic rights, and like him they too frequently regret the bargain. Their enlistment is no doubt voluntary, but not so with their service, which is a long one, and looked upon by the soldier as a life-time. The price to pay for his liberty is beyond his reach ; so if discontented and unhappy, he often breaks the contract. This leads to individual suffering and great less to the state. It is in a measure being deprived of a high order of independence, known only perhaps to themselves and the American citizen, that makes the recruit inclined to resist the restraint which is so closely wound round him, and modern recruits also feel the worry or annoyances of discipline far more keenly than their fathers did. There is an anxiety attendant on military life, though not of a pecuniary nature, which for the first few years, especially until the man is moulded into a proper groove and thoroughly knows what he is about, produces a constant nervous strain of a description unknown in civil life. Whether at home or abroad, the soldier is subjected

to this ; there is no immunity from it, and we have before seen
how directly all this reacts on the heart.   I fear the system of
keeping men constantly employed about trifles "to keep them
out of mischief," is not a wholesome one, for objectless labour is a
depressing punishment.   Moreover, such employment as routine
or ordinary duties is not of an invigorating nature, although there
is some rivalry and emulation connected with it.   For the most part
it devolves into a rather monotonous struggle to keep up to the
mark and out of scrapes.   Thus the anxiety is of a strangely depressing nature, to look out for one's self, and see what next is
likely to arise, and while thus always on the alert, there is no
care for the morrow ; he feels that he is at the mercy of the
state, he cannot add to his individual comforts, clothing, or ne-
cessaries ; thus it is he becomes reckless and careless of events.
Few anxieties in civil life are accompanied by the same tendency
to act in a depressing manner on the feelings.   With the soldier they are such that the most he can expect is to get off free,
and if punished he can scarce hope to recoup the loss of a sen-
tence ; he knows and feels it is recorded against him during ·his
entire career.   It is to be feared many uneducated privates
are not calculating enough to see the bright side that undoubtedly exists.   Again, the struggle in civil life among the soldier's
class is far different.   Here it is for the maintenance of the individual, to add to his material comforts ; or the man works that
good may come of it to his wife or offspring.   The other, cut off
from all home ties, works solely for the benefit of the state.
Thus the impetus that stimulates his labours is of very different
nature.   Although much of late has been done that tends to
make men thrifty and careful, still, more hope and opportunity
of benefiting himself, more individuality and self-reliance, are
required.   There can be little doubt but there are a recklessness
of character, an unwholesome anxiety and constant nervous
strain, brought on by military life, which create a morbid
desire for drink, and possibly predispose to *delirium tremens* or
other mental affections.   It is quite probable that there is less
drunkenness in the army than among the soldier's class in civil

life, because it is watched over, and the means taken to check it are prompt and severe ; but I believe, from the above and various other causes, there is a greater craving for liquor among soldiers. Drink leads to prison, and in the effects of prison regime, to which our soldiers are subjected to a far greater extent than the civil community, may be discovered another source from which springs that nervous derangement of their hearts. Misdemeanors, not in themselves of a vicious nature, or offences against the criminal law that would scarce engage the attention of civil functionaries, may be treated as of a very serious character when adjudicated on by military law as offences against the Mutiny Act or Articles of War. It is young soldiers for the most part that get into trouble, and desertions among these men alone would increase the average of comparison considerably, owing to the punishments consequent on their desertion. And here we may find a fertile source of cardiac affections ; for by depressing the vital powers, mental and bodily, the deranged portion of the frame, or that most continually or strongly acted on, will be the first to give way. In prison the feelings are suppressed and the mind strongly affected, consequently, in very many instances, after a course of prison life, men have to be taken into hospital, fed up, and rested, until the heart regains its equilibrium. Medical officers of civil prisons who deal with the criminal classes must carefully guard against the impositions of those who would try to evade justice or the severity of the punishment awarded ; but those who are accustomed to deal with soldiers and the keeping of them in health in the interests of the state, must take a broad view of the matter. Here the health of the soldier should be the first consideration. Army surgeons are for many reasons unfavourably disposed to grant any indulgence to men who "commit themselves"—they will be no party to the common and too truthful expression, " That fellow is always either in jail or in hospital." That health is unfavourably affected by prison is recognized in the *Gymnastic Instructions*, for men from prison are treated as weakly men recovering from illness, by placing them in the same category. It is wisely laid down:—"That men out from hospital or prison ought to be certified as fit for instruction." It may be said, judging from statistics of the average daily strength and admissions to hospital, that men in prison "enjoy" better health than their comrades in the same garrison; yet there are certain disabilities, the effects of dissipation, or conviviality, or minor accidents, to which men in prison are not liable, and it must be remembered that they are practically sound when sent to prison; they are for the most part young men, and as a rule only in for short periods. While in prison they would not be admitted on account of trivial complaints; it is when they come out of prison they go into hospital; but I merely draw attention to prison life as one of those incidental causes which tend to increase the average, and stamp the peculiarity of cardiac affections in the service, although it may otherwise affect men as regards phthisis or mental derangements.

In addition to the two per cent. said to be always in prison (this is rather a high average, for it seems there are under 11,000 soldiers daily in jail at home), there are a great number of minor offences, which come under the jurisdiction of commanding officers, dealt with regimentally, such, for instance, as are punished by confinements to barracks, defaulter's drill, and cells up to seven days. Perhaps it would be more within the mark to say that two per cent. of the army are daily undergoing some form of these punishments, than that they are in garrison prisons. Yet even the comparatively trivial matter of confining men in the guard-room, with the subsequent bringing up, weighing off, or letting off with a caution, are all harassing and health-destroying, and if of no immediate injury, they undoubtedly tend to wear out and age men; while it is on the nervous centres, and consequently on the heart, that the full brunt of them falls. It is not easy to say to what degree these influences are felt; they differ in regiments; but such conditions must tend to depress the vital powers, and induce that nervous exhaustion of an irritative type recorded as palpitation.

"Discipline," the *World* says, "is to an army very much what jelly is to a pie—a firm, yet not an entirely rigid and unyielding bond, whereby many heterogeneous constituents are held together in one solid and compact mass. No considerable body of men can be governed and manipulated without it; through it and by it alone can be obtained that prompt obedience, that unhesitating submission and subordination of will, that unity of action, upon which the value and efficiency of an army primarily depend. It is a law alike to officers and men: old soldiers will conform to it almost automatically; if the young chafe at it at first, ere long, when sufficiently subjected to it, habit becomes second nature also with them. It must be judiciously administered—intelligently, yet without undue relaxation. . . . . The soldier is still circumscribed by many childish restrictions: no schoolboy suffers more irksome restraints upon his liberty and his time. Confined to barracks until a certain hour of the day, forbidden to wander more than a mile or two from camp or cantonment, or, without special previous permission, to remain absent after a certain hour of the night, subjected on his return to needlessly minute inspections to detect the slightest taint of vicious excitement, his temper is apt to be yet further soured by a repressive system, short-sighted and inelastic, which makes mountains out of molehills and magnifies small *lâches* into heinous crimes. More vexatious and physically unpleasant is the stupid practice which still largely prevails of relegating soldiers to the guard-room for even trivial offences; thus condemning them for a silly speech or a slight difference of opinion with a superior, for temporary accidental absence or slight neglect of duty, to loss of bed for the night, and the enforced companionship in a repulsive prison of comrades the most drunken and disreputable. There are yet again the constantly recurring petty annoyances endured at the hands of tyrants great and small—of coarsely upbraiding drill-corporal, of overbearing pay-sergeant, unscrupulous for his own ends, of captain, fastidious to madness over such trifles as the fit of accoutrements or personal bearing and carriage, or, last of all, of zealous domineering colonel, who has fixed his standard of efficiency at so high a level that, although assiduously aimed at by harassing drills and incessant parades, it is never actually attained."

Although here the criticism is rather too severe, I think it well to direct the attention of medical officers to it, more especially as they have now gained a position of independence from which they can impartially observe such matters.

Discipline, then, is the chief thing that deprives hygienic conditions of their invigorating power, develops certain cardiac affections, and renders our army, and probably others also, as unhealthy as they are. Much the same may be said of parade work; for on account of the conditions under which it is carried on, which have been before alluded to, it is deprived of what it otherwise would be—a healthy and invigorating out-door exercise. Sir J. Ronald Martin wrote :—"What 'the interior discipline and economy' of Marlborough, England's greatest commander, may have been, I have no means of knowing; but there must have been something notable in that order which, according to one who served under him, made his camp resemble 'a well-governed city. Cursing and swearing were seldom heard among the officers ; a sot and a drunkard was the object of scorn ; and the poor soldiers, many of them the refuse and dregs of the nation, became, at the close of one or two campaigns, tractable, civil, sensible, and clean, and had an air and spirit above the vulgar.' Such results were worthy 'the head of European captains,' as Napoleon termed him ; but how melancholy to look on the reverse of this picture, and to reflect that in the middle of the nineteenth century so much should remain to be done to render the British soldier healthy and happy. On the abuse of ardent spirits in our various colonies it were almost in vain to speak. Before that terrible vice can be overcome, something far more powerful than medical reasoning on facts, or the warnings of experience founded on them, must be brought into active operation. Discipline must still further alter its direction. In place of being active only to punish wrong, it ought and must be exerted further and further in the encouragement to good conduct."

As well as those altered circumstances, by which the soldier is surrounded in his new career, and those punishments to which he is liable by living under military law, the operation of which on their own persons few can ever hope to escape, there is another incidental condition, namely, foreign service, which, in addition to its baneful influences on the constitution generally, grants no protection as regards heart affections. Of foreign countries, India, both by reason of number of men there, and the nature of the diseases of its climate, is by far the most formidable enemy in this shape the British soldier has to encounter. Out of the United Kingdom, cavalry, horse, and field artillery are only liable to take service in India, and these men are seldom or never stationed out of the plains; they only go to the hills when invalided, to convalescent depôts. The infantry and a few garrison artillery occupy hill stations; this difference of residence, combined with the nature of their several employments, will account for the comparative difference in the heart affections of these arms of the service at home and in India. In round numbers, two-thirds of our cavalry and horse artillery are serving in the plains of India; and half the infantry stationed in that country are quartered in the hills—located, it appears, in situations unfavourable to the production of either heart disease or rheumatism. Now from the following figures may arise the question whether it is the infantry make these stations show a comparative immunity from disease, or whether the climate and other conditions acting on them make this favourable difference? I believe the latter to be the case. I abstract the following from Mr. Myers's valuable essay, so frequently referred to:—"The following statistics show what little difference there is in the deaths from heart disease in the three chief divisions of the service in this country, and the slight excess in the invaliding for the same in the infantry.

"Diseases of circulatory system in three arms of the United Kingdom, excluding household cavalry and depôts, 1860 to 1866, inclusive :—

	Strength.	Died.	Ratio per 1,000.	Invalided.	Ratio per 1,000.
Cavalry, ...	62,117	50	·80	234	3·91
Artillery, ...	63,176	56	·88	223	3·52
Infantry, ...	168,385	144	·80	891	4.37

"According to Dr. Bryden's tables (vide *Indian Medical Gazette*, May 1st, 1869) the reverse holds good in India, thus:—

HEART DISEASE AND ANEURISM DURING THREE YEARS, 1865 TO 1867.

	Ratio of deaths per 1,000.	Ratio of invaliding per 1,000.
Cavalry, ...	2·06	4.90
Artillery, ...	.86	4.33
Infantry, ...	.90	2.63

"Statistics of heart disease in India must, however, show great variation, according to circumstances, as was shown in a very able article on the subject, published in the *Standard* of March 27th, 1869, and from which the following is extracted :—'The highest ratio of mortality from diseases of the circulatory system in Bengal in 1866, viz., 3·46, occurred amongst the troops who are reported 'on the march;' and an almost identical result is shown by an examination of the Bombay army in 1866 ; for, whilst the death-rate from diseases of the organs of circulation of the total force (12,077) was only ·66, that of the troops on the march was 3·38 per 1,000—a very striking fact.

"Dr. Bryden's statistical table, however, clearly proves that in India the cavalry and artillery suffer more from these diseases than the infantry; and such is the invariable opinion of the many army medical officers who have kindly given me their personal experiences." In the infantry, rapidity of movements in camps at home at uncertain periods, and autumn manœuvres, while their employments are probably not so interesting or allowing of so much individual freedom of action as those

employed about horses, may account for the difference here
stated. Musketry or rifle practice, which occupies so much
time in the infantry, is far more of a parade than stable duties.
Everyone acquainted with marching in India must know, when
compared with a sedentary life in cantonments, that it will tend to
develop latent disability.

As well as the great number of invalids sent. home annually
on account of heart affections, it seems that nearly one-half
the total number invalided are returned under the head
of "General Debility." Now I would venture to say, from
my own experience, that in a very great many of these
instances the heart has been deranged, although perhaps not
the prominent feature of the case. Thus it is very difficult
to ascertain how far this disease ramifies through the army, and
to what extent it may be developed by service in India, where
it is quite as common, if not more so, than at home. In the
Blue Book for 1875, once before referred to, we read, for " *debility*
one-third more men were invalided from Bengal than in 1874.
No explanation is apparent for the large increase in the number of men sent to England on account of a condition for reco-
very from which it might be imagined that a residence at a hill
station in the country was especially likely to be sufficient."
This strengthens the opinion stated from what I observed in the
East.

The depressing effects of climate and malarial poisons, acting
on those predisposed or affected with latent disability, give rise to
so-called cardiac dyspepsia, nervous exhaustion, or irritability of
heart; or again, in some instances, in combination with other
causes, the heart's action may be interfered with by displacements, on account of liver and splenic enlargements ; but the
counterbalancing influences which preserve the ratio of quality
between the United Kingdom and the East, are the amount of
relaxation, and absence of worry and anxiety, attendant on
duties in the latter place, as well as the change of dress, which
relieves men from all restrictions in this respect. Yet, as regards
dress, the infantry who occupy the hill stations are the only

men who wear their English tunics during the greater part of the year, and we see how comparatively free from heart affections they are in India. Men in the plains wear loose serge or white drill patrol jackets.

I have not the means by me of knowing, but suppose about 1,400 men have been invalided home from India during the last five years on account of diseases of the circulatory system—that is to say, men absolutely affected, as shown by statistics; and from 1863 to 1867, according to Myers's tables, 1,346 have been invalided out of the service. What the expense to the state this amount of disease must be directly, can perhaps be ascertained with tolerable accuracy ; but what the effect on recruiting this number of, for the most part young men, being sent back to their homes after a short absence, either permanently incapacitated from hard work, or in a dying condition, is not easy to fully comprehend. The effect must be great indeed, and bears strongly on one of the most important questions that can engage the attention of the Legislature.

I have looked all round, as far as my knowledge and present means of obtaining information extends, and cannot find a hitch anywhere as to the correctness of these views of the causation of the excessive amount of disease of the circulatory system met with in the army. While endeavouring to bring matters plainly forward, it was at the same time necessary to point out how inadequate are what may be called the received ideas to account for the amount of disease, and the special form it assumes, when developed in and by the service.

Can this excess of disease be prevented ? I believe only in a degree. It can only be reduced so as to approximate more towards what has been observed in civil life ; the average will always be high, on account of the necessary restrictions of discipline, as well as those incidental conditions connected with our soldier's career. But if correct as to its causation, the means to be taken for its mitigation are self-evident. In addition to those affections induced by general causes, to which the hearts of all men are liable, the soldiers, we see, are acted on by special

causes; such as causes acting mechanically, either directly or
indirectly interfering with the arrangements of the heart and
great vessels, and those which act or react on the heart through
the nervous centres.   In suggesting remedies for the mitigation
or prevention of diseases of the circulatory system, attention
should be principally directed to the special causes, particularly
those in connection with the physical training and teaching of
subordination to young men, as well as the mode of conducting
duties, internal economy, and discipline.   There are such a
combination of circumstances set at work at the same time, while
teaching and remodelling the man, and so connected are they
together—so perfect is the system—that it would be extremely
difficult to separate them, or trace the tendency or effects of each.
So, taken as they are collectively, we may say it is our military
system and conditions of service that induce this class of affections, and not any one cause, such as certain diseases, vicious
habits, constitutional infirmity, dress, alcohol, tobacco, coffee,
quinine, or excessive work.   Nor are these, all taken together,
sufficient, without mental influences, to account for the preponderance and speciality of affections of the circulatory system
which occurs in the army.

It seems the system might be improved by allowing more
time for the setting-up, position drill, and training of the soldier.
No matter what his age may be, he should not be subjected to
any sudden or violent alteration of his natural shape, and in this
manner have his heart and lungs directly interfered with.
Perchance this sudden alteration of the shape of the chest
may account for some of the "phthisis" which occurs in the
service.   Tubercular deposits in the soldier frequently begin in
the upper portion of the right lung; in the civilian the left is
more frequently first affected.   The liver is on the right side,
and this gland descends with the diaphragm considerably during
the alteration of the shape of the thorax, as before described.
Thus the upper portion of the right lung, having lost support,
may possibly be exposed to injury by over-distension to fill the
vacuum.   It is more likely to be thus affected than by external

compression ; for in the infantry a heavy pouch-belt presses over the apex of the left lung, yet "the mortality from tuberculosus in the infantry of the line, is below the mean mortality of the army at large."—*Parkes.*

In expanding the chest, such powerful instruments as dumb-bells ought not to be used ; " while the heart and lungs ought to be educated, so to speak," in order that the most immediately concerned organs may be prepared for any unusual or unaccus-tomed work they may be called upon to do. I have referred to parade work to show that for the most part it is not of an invigorating nature, owing to the conditions under which it is carried on, while it is also considered insufficient for the physical requirements of the soldier. But the gymnasium is well suited to supply this want; still it ought to be extended more, and made as little as possible of a parade. In a convenient spot close by every barracks, under a tree or shed, some fixed apparatus ought to be put up, such as a horizontal bar and mock horse, where men who felt so inclined could go of their own free will, and practice. To relieve as much as possible anxieties, the mental faculties of those newly joined ought to be carefully dealt with, and not unduly excited through worry, bewilder-ment, or vexation. While off duty, men ought to be granted, as far as can be, rest not liable to interference, to establish a feeling of freedom when their work is over.

I may again add that the great physiologist, Claud Bernard, repeatedly asserts—and this deserves special notice—" that when the heart is affected it reacts on the brain, and the state of the brain, again, reacts through the pneumogastric-nerve on the heart, so that under any excitement there will be much mutual action and reaction between these, the two most important organs of the body." If men are uncomfortable they soon become discontented, and their duties feel irksome or monotonous, and this, with the constant surveillance and various conditions to which they are subjected, too frequently causes men to become reckless and careless ; and this character, together with a parti-ality for drink, is so often developed, that the discharged soldier is generally looked upon as a worthless member of society.

Although things are advancing, and men will be taught to be somewhat thrifty and careful in the future, still something more might be done to improve their present condition, and add to their individual comforts, so that they may be happy and contented and feel at home in the service, while making a provision for the future. Undoubtedly it is the young soldier feels restraint most, and also those anxieties attendant on his duties, while at the same time home-ties are still fresh in his memory; and although in this respect, distance may lend enchantment to the view, still the feeling is there, and ought to be counteracted by making barrack-rooms more homely. One of the first things to do in this way is to fit up the walls of barrack-rooms with small cupboards, one for each man, to have two keys, one with the man, the other with the officer commanding his company. Here the soldier would have a place to lay by many little articles of comfort—his letters, photographs, pipe, watch, or book, or a candle to read by in the dimly-lit-up room, also unmarked articles of uniform may be left there. Now the way things are concealed or kept out of sight is certainly not comfortable, although the room looks trim, and according to orders. I have seen in a man-of-war, small boxes, not regulation, permitted, for each blue-jacket and marine—simple boxes, fitted up with an ink bottle only, and to see all the little knick-knacks they stowed away in these was really surprising. Barrack-room cupboards may be objected to on the grounds that they would become receptacles for rubbish and liquor; but not so with proper supervision, while the expense of these fittings, and the transport of such articles as would probably result from this arrangement, would be a mere bagatelle, compared with the comfort, contentment, and happiness it would bestow on the army. At the same time nothing would convey to the mind of the soldier more forcibly the idea that he was cared for, not collectively but individually and directly, for it would take no mental effort to understand the intention. His physical comforts, his surroundings, and belongings would point it out, and bring the matter home to him. Now a man is obliged to live without feeling the benefit of any such advantages, save those conferred by a regulation kit. Perhaps in accordance with this arrangement, he is supposed to be ready to take the field at a moment's notice; but as a counterbalancing effect of the application of this principle, we see that the soldier is no doubt bereft of many personal or home comforts, almost essential to his well-being, or the development of that vigour without which you cannot have perfect efficiency. These things bear on a question asked by Parkes : " How is a soldier to be made not merely healthy and vigorous, but courageous, hopeful, and enduring ? "

Improvements have been made in the infantry soldier's dress; but he has not enough of changes for broken weather. The so-called stable jacket, which is, by the way, never worn at stables, I hope will soon be discontinued, as it seems a most worthless article of dress. A casual observer seeing a party of men in cold, draughty stables, or walking to and from their barrack-rooms in shirt-sleeves during the depths of winter, while labourers are wrapped up in comforters and warm waistcoats, might fancy such exposure due to the " proverbial recklessness of the British soldier." Not so; it lies in this : the man's clothes are unsuited to his work, while his surroundings have a tendency rather to perpetuate the saying. A good deal of the soldier's illness may be traced to imperfections in clothing. But with respect to diseases of the circulatory system, I have sufficiently pointed out that it cannot be the cause of so much disease as we have. Of course instances may occur in which it is the starting point; but as a rule the dress of a soldier is merely an accessory cause, acting in conjunction with many others of its class. The comfort and suitability of dress is of course a matter of the greatest importance. Just look at a party of blue-jackets at gun-drill, and contrast their serviceable dress with that of garrison artillery in tight useless jackets, that have to be thrown aside before the men can work. It is not the amount of work that affects the soldier, or wears him out quicker than the civilian. Give him plenty of exercise in the way of physical labour at regular periods, but with equivalent hours of relaxation. From the commencement, induce the soldier to look upon the service more as a home where all his wants are supplied; but we must study his wants more closely, and supply remedies for the prevention of such weaknesses or peculiarities of his character as are at present developed by the service. If this were done, we should have more of that contentment and happiness which is so conducive to good health, and perhaps shall hear less about competition with the labour market for men. For there are attractions, if developed, in connection with military life—bands and uniform—that put a mere rate of pay calculation out of the question. For no mercantile establishment could supply anything equivalent in competition.

I hope my province has not been overstepped while touching on some of those almost essentially military matters, which may be considered, as it were, outside the pale of hygienic conditions; but there are some imperfections in our system which, if judiciously corrected, where the principle is sound, will be health-improving and invigorating, and, above all, tend to reduce the amount of that costly class of affections we have been considering.

THE END.

R. D. WEBB AND SON, PRINTERS, DUBLIN.

WORKS

PUBLISHED BY

FANNIN AND CO.

41, GRAFTON-STREET, DUBLIN.

Supplied in London by

LONGMANS, GREEN & CO.; SIMPKIN, MARSHALL & CO.
EDINBURGH: MACLACHLAN AND STEWART.
MELBOURNE: GEORGE ROBERTSON.

A Treatise on Rheumatic Gout, or Chronic Rheumatic Arthritis of all the Joints.

Illustrated by Woodcuts and an Atlas of Plates. By ROBERT ADAMS, M.D., Fellow and Ex-President of the Royal College of Surgeons in Ireland: formerly Surgeon to the Richmond Hospital; and Surgeon in Ordinary to the Queen in Ireland, etc. 8vo. and 4to. Atlas. Second edition. 21s.

Clinical Lectures on Diseases Peculiar to Women.

By LOOMBE ATTHILL, M.D. (Univ. Dub.), Fellow and Examiner in Midwifery, King and Queen's College of Physicians; Master of the Dublin Lying-in Hospital. Fourth edition, post 8vo. [In the Press.

Medical Education and Medical Interests.

Carmichael Prize Essay. By ISAAC ASHE, M.D. M.Ch. Univ. Dub., Physician-Superintendent, Dundrum Central Asylum for the Insane, Ireland. 165 pp. 4s.

By the same Author:

Medical Politics:

Being the Essay to which was awarded the First Carmichael Prize of £200, by the Council of the Royal College of Surgeons, Ireland, 1873. Crown 8vo.f 174 pp., cloth. 4s.

The Pathology and Treatment of Syphilis, Chancroid Ulcers, and their Complications.

By JOHN K. BARTON, M.D. (Dub.) F.R.C.S.I. ; Surgeon to the Adelaide Hospital ; Lecturer on Surgery, Ledwich School of Medicine ; Visiting Surgeon, Convalescent Home, Stillorgan. 8vo. 306 pp. 7s.

Contributions to Medicine and Midwifery.

By THOMAS EDWARD BEATTY, M.D. T.C.D:, F.K. & Q.C.P. ; late President of the King and Queen's College of Physicians in Ireland. 8vo., Illustrated with Lithographic Plates, coloured and plain, 651 pp. 15s., reduced to 8s.

Essays and Reports on Operative and Conservative Surgery.

By RICHARD G. BUTCHER, F.R.C.S.I. ; M.D. Dub. ; Lecturer on Operative and Practical Surgery to Sir P. Dun's Hospital ; Examiner in Surgery, University of Dublin ; etc. Illustrated by 62 Lithographic Plates, coloured and plain ; and several Engravings on Wood. 8vo. cloth. 21s.

A Treatise on Disease of the Heart.

By O'BRYEN BELLINGHAM, M.D., F.R.C.S.I. ; late Surgeon to St. Vincent's Hospital, etc. 8vo., 621 pp., cloth. 6s.

Clinical Lectures on Venereal Diseases.

By RICHARD CARMICHAEL, F.R.C.S. ; late Consulting Surgeon to the Richmond, Hardwicke, and Whitworth Hospitals, etc. 8vo., with Coloured Plates. 7s. 6d., reduced to 2s. 6d.

On the Theory and Practice of Midwifery.

By FLEETWOOD CHURCHILL, M.D., Fellow and Ex-President of the King and Queen's College of Physicians; formerly Professor of Midwifery to the King and Queen's College of Physicians. Sixth edition, corrected and enlarged, illustrated by 119 highly finished Wood Engravings. Foolscap 8vo., cloth. 12s. 6d.

By the same Author :

A Manual for Midwives and Nurses.

Third edition. Foolscap 8vo., cloth. 4s.

By the same Author:

The Diseases of Children.

Third edition, revised and enlarged. Post 8vo., 900 pp. 12s. 6d.

By the same Author:

On the Diseases of Women, including those of Pregnancy and Childbed.

Sixth edition, corrected and enlarged. Illustrated by 57 Engravings on Wood. Post 8vo., cloth. 15s.

A Dictionary of Practical Surgery and Encyclopædia of Surgical Science.

By SAMUEL COOPER, F.R C.S.; late Senior Surgeon to the University College Hospital, and Professor of Surgery in University College. New edition, brought down to the present time by SAMUEL A. LANE, Surgeon to St. Mary's, and Consulting Surgeon to the Lock Hospitals; Lecturer on Surgery at St. Mary's Hospital; assisted by various eminent Surgeons. 8vo., 2 vols. £2 10s.

Manual of the Medicinal Preparations of Iron,

Including their Preparation, Chemistry, Physiological Action, and Therapeutic Use, with an Appendix containing the Iron Preparations of the British Pharmacopœia. By HARRY NAPIER DRAPER, F.C.S. Post 8vo., cloth. 2s. 6d.

The Dublin Dissector, or System of Practical Anatomy.

By ROBERT HARRISON, F.R.C.S.; formerly Professor of Anatomy in the University of Dublin. Fifth edition. 2 vols., foolscap 8vo. Illustrated with 160 Wood Engravings. 12s. 6d.

The Dublin Journal of Medical Science,

Containing original Communications, Reviews, Abstracts, and Reports in Medicine, Surgery, and the Collateral Sciences. Published monthly. Subscription £1 per annum, delivered free in all places within the range of the British book post, if paid for in advance.

Proceedings of the Dublin Obstetrical Society

For Sessions 1871-'72; 1872-'73; 1873-'74; 1874-'75. 8vo., cloth. 5s. each volume.

The Personal Responsibility of the Insane.

By JAMES F. DUNCAN, M.D. (Dub.); Fellow and Ex-President, King and Queen's College of Physicians, etc. Post 8vo., cloth, 3s.

By the same Author:

Popular Errors on Insanity Examined and Exposed.

Foolscap 8vo., cloth, 265 pp. 4s. 6d.

Physiological Remarks upon the Causes of Consumption.

By VALENTINE DUKE, M.D., F.R.C.S. 8vo., cloth. 3s. 6d.

By the same Author:

An Essay on the Cerebral Affections of Children:

Being the Council Prize Essay awarded by the Provincial Medical and Surgical Association. 8vo., cloth. 8s.

The Ophthalmoscopic Appearances of the Optic Nerve in cases of Cerebral Tumour.

By C. E. FITZGERALD, M.D. Ch.M. (Dub.); Ophthalmic Surgeon to the Richmond Hospital; Surgeon-Oculist to the Queen in Ireland: Assistant-Surgeon to the National Eye and Ear Infirmary; Lecturer on Ophthalmic Surgery, Carmichael School of Medicine. 8vo., with Coloured Plates. 1s. 6d.

Elements of Matoria Medica,

Containing the Chemistry and Natural History of Drugs, their Effects, Doses, and Adulteration. By DR. WILLIAM FRASER, Lecturer on Materia Medica to Carmichael School of Medicine. 8vo., 453 pp. 10s. 6d.

By the same Author:

Treatment of Diseases of the Skin.

Foolscap 8vo., 174 pp. 3s.

On the Origin of Species by means of Organic Affinity.

By H. FREKE, M.D., F.K. & Q.C.P. ; Physician to Dr. Steevens's Hospital ; Lecturer on the Practice of Physic and Clinical Medicine in Steevens's Hospital School of Medicine. 8vo., cloth. 5s.

Remarks on the Prevalence and Distribution of Fever in Dublin.

By THOMAS W. GRIMSHAW, M.D. (Dub. Univ.) ; Fellow and Censor of the King and Queen's College of Physicians ; Physician to Dr. Steevens's Hospital and to Cork-street Fever Hospital, Dublin. Illustrated by a Map, Tables, and Diagrams, with Appendices on Sanitary matters in that City. 8vo. 1s.

A System of Botanical Analysis,

Applied to the Diagnosis of British Natural Orders. By W. HANDSEL GRIFFITHS, PH.D., L.R.C.P., L.R.C.S. Edin. ; Lecturer on Chemistry in the Ledwich School of Medicine, Dublin ; etc. For the use of beginners. 8vo. 1s. 6d.

By the same Author :

Notes on the Pharmacopœial Preparations,

Specially arranged for the use of Students preparing for examination. Post 8vo. 2s. 6d.

By the same Author :

Posological Tables :

A Classified Chart of Doses. Intended for Students as an aid to memory, and for Practitioners, Prescribers, and Dispensers, as a work of Reference. 1s.

The Present State of the Army Medical Service as a Life Career for the Surgeon.

By EDWARD HAMILTON, M.D. (Dub.) ; Fellow and Ex-President of the Royal College of Surgeons in Ireland ; one of the Surgeons to Dr. Steevens's Hospital, and Lecturer on Anatomy and Physiology in the Medical School, etc. Royal 8vo. 1s. 6d.

The Restoration of a Lest Nose by Operation.

By JOHN HAMILTON, F.R.C.S.I.; late Surgeon to the Queen in Ireland; formerly Surgeon to the Richmond Hospital; and Surgeon to St. Patrick's Hospital for Lunatics, etc. Illustrated with Wood Engravings. 8vo. 2s.

By the same Author:

Essays on Syphilis.

Essay I.—Syphilitic Sarcocele. 8vo., with Coloured Plates. 2s. 6d

By the same Author:

Lectures on Syphilitic Osteitis and Periostitis.

8vo., cloth, 108 pp., with 12 Illustrations, some Coloured. 5s.

The Diseases of the Heart and of the Aorta.

By THOMAS HAYDEN, F.K. & Q.C.P.; Physician to the Mater Misericordiæ Hospital; Professor of Anatomy and Physiology in the Catholic University of Dublin; etc. 8vo., 1,232 pp., with 80 Illustrations on Wood and Steel. 25s.

Report on the Cholera Epidemic of 1866,

As treated in the Mater Misericordiæ Hospital; with General Remarks on the Disease. Revised and reprinted from the Dublin Quarterly Journal of Medical Science, May, 1867. By THOMAS HAYDEN, M.D., Fellow K. & Q.C.P., etc; and F. R. CRUISE, M.D. (Dub.); F.K. & Q.C.P.; Physicians to the Hospital. Royal 8vo. 1s.

On Diseases of the Prostate Gland.

By JAMES STANNUS HUGHES, M.D., F.R.C.S.I.; Surgeon to Jervis-street Hospital; Professor of Surgery in the Royal College of Surgeons. Illustrated with Plates. Second edition, foolscap 8vo., cloth, 3s.

By the same Author:

Œdema of the Glottis:

Its Clinical History, Pathology, and Treatment. 1s.

Hooper's Physician's Vade Mecum;

A Manual of the Principles and Practice of Physic, with an Outline of General Pathology, Therapeutics, and Hygiene. Ninth edition, revised by WILLIAM AUGUSTUS GUY, M.B., F.R.C.S. (Cantab.), and JOHN HARLEY, M.D., F.L.S., F.R.C.P. (Lond.) Foolscap 8vo., 688 pp., cloth. 12s. 6d.

The Study of Life.

By H. MacNaughton Jones, M.D., Ch.M., Fellow of the Royal College of Surgeons, Ireland and Edinburgh; etc. 8vo., 80 pp. 1s. 6d.

Hospitalism and Zymotic Diseases, as more especially illustrated by Puerperal Fever, or Metria;

A Paper read in the Hall of the College of Physicians. By Evory Kennedy, M.D. (Edin. and Dub.) ; Fellow and Ex-President of the King and Queen's College of Physicians ; Past President of the Obstetrical Society ; Ex-Master of the Dublin Lying-in Hospital. Also a Reply to the Criticisms of Seventeen Physicians upon this Paper. Second edition, royal 8vo., 132 pp., cloth. 5s.

Some Account of the Epidemic of Scarlatina

which prevailed in Dublin from 1834 to 1842, inclusive, with Observations. By Henry Kennedy, M.B., F.K. & Q.C.P. ; Physician to the Cork-street Fever Hospital. Foolscap 8vo., cloth. 4s. 6d.

Observations on Venereal Diseases,

Derived from Civil and Military Practice. By Hamilton Labatt, F.R.C.S. Post 8vo., cloth. 6s. 6d.

The Practical and Descriptive Anatomy of the Human Body.

By Thomas H. Ledwich, F.R.C.S. ; late Surgeon to the Meath Hospital ; and Lecturer on Anatomy and Physiology in the Ledwich School of Medicine; and Edward Ledwich, F.R.C.S., Surgeon to Mercer's Hospital ; Lecturer on Anatomy and Physiology in the Ledwich School of Medicine. Second edition. Post 8vo., cloth. 12s. 6d.

Clinical Memoirs on Diseases of Women:

Being the results of Eleven Years' experience in the Gynecological Wards of the Dublin Lying-in Hospital. By Alfred H. M'Clintock, M.D., F.R.C.S. ; late Master of the Dublin Lying-in Hospital ; Honorary Fellow of the Obstetrical Society of London, etc. Illustrated with 35 Wood Engravings, 8vo., cloth, 449 pp. 12s. 6d.

Lectures and Essays on the Science and Practice of Surgery.

Part I.—Lectures on Venereal Disease. Part II.—The Physiology and Pathology of the Spinal Cord. By Robert M'Donnell, M.D., F.R.S. ; Fellow and Member of the Court of Examiners, Royal College of Surgeons in Ireland ; one of the Surgeons to Dr. Steevens's Hospital, etc. 8vo., 2s. 6d. each part.

By the same Author :

Observations on the Functions of the Liver.

8vo., 38 pp. 1s.

Botanical Companion to the British Pharmacopœia.

By Hyman Marks, L.R.C.S.I. 8vo. 1s.

The Presence of Organic Matter in Potable Water always deleterious to Health;

to which is added the Modern Analysis. By O'Brien Mahony, L.R.C.P. (Edin.), etc. Second edition, 8vo. 2s. 6d.

A Manual of Physiology and of the Principles of Disease ;

To which is added over 1,000 Questions by the Author, and selected from those of Examining Bodies ; and a Glossary of Medical Terms. By E. D. Mapother, M.D. ; Fellow and Professor of Anatomy and Physiology, Royal College of Surgeons ; Surgeon to St. Vincent's Hospital. Second edition, foolscap 8vo., 566 pp., with 150 Illustrations. 10s. 6d.

By the same Author :

Lectures on Public Health,

Delivered at the Royal College of Surgeons. Second edition, with numerous Illustrations. Foolscap 8vo. 6s.

By the same Author :

FIRST CARMICHAEL PRIZE ESSAY.

The Medical Profession and its Educational and Licensing Bodies.

The circumstances of the various branches of Medical Practice, as well as of the Modes of Education and Examination, are described, in order to make the work useful to those choosing a profession. Foolscap 8vo., 227 pp. 5s.

By the same Author :

Lectures on Skin Diseases,

Delivered at St. Vincent's Hospital. Second edition, 212 pp., with Illustrations. 3s. 6d.

Neligan's Medicines: their Uses and Mode of Administration;

Including a Complete Conspectus of the British Pharmacopœia, an account of New Remedies, and an Appendix of Formulæ. By DR. RAWDON MACNAMARA, Professor of Materia Medica, Royal College of Surgeons in Ireland ; Surgeon to the Meath Hospital ; Examiner in Materia Medica, University of Dublin, etc. Seventh edition, 8vo., cloth, 934 pp. 18s.

An Atlas of Cutaneous Diseases;

Containing nearly 100 Coloured Illustrations of Skin Diseases. By DR. J. MOORE NELIGAN. Small folio, half bound in leather. 25s., reduced to 17s. 6d.

By the same Author :

A Practical Treatise on Diseases of the Skin.

Second edition, revised and enlarged by T. W. BELCHER, M.D. (Dub.); Fellow of King and Queen's College of Physicians in Ireland, formerly Physician to the Dublin Dispensary for Skin Diseases, etc. Post 8vo. 6s.

Anatomy of the Arteries of the Human Body,

Descriptive and Surgical, with the Descriptive Anatomy of the Heart. By JOHN HATCH POWER, M.D., F.R.C.S., formerly Professor of Surgery in the Royal College of Surgeons ; Surgeon to the City of Dublin Hospital. New edition, with illustrations from Drawings made expressly for this work by B. W. Richardson, F.R.C.S., Surgeon to the Adelaide Hospital, etc. Foolscap 8vo., cloth. Plain, 10s. 6d. ; Coloured, 12s.

Nature and Treatment of Deformities of the Human Body;

Being a course of Lectures delivered at the Meath Hospital, Dublin. By LAMBERT H. ORMSBY, M.B. (Univ. Dub.) ; F.R.C.S.I.; Surgeon to the Meath Hospital and County Dublin Infirmary, etc. Post 8vo., illustrated with Wood Engravings. 263 pp. 5s.

A Manual of Public Health for Ireland,

For the use of Members of Sanitary Authorities, Officers of Health, and Students of State Medicine. By THOMAS W. GRIMSHAW, M.D. M.A., Diplomate in State Medicine of Trin. Coll. Dublin ; Physician to Cork-street (Fever) and Steevens's Hospitals ; J. EMERSON REYNOLDS, M.D. F.C.S., Professor of Chemistry, University of Dublin ; ROBERT O'B. FURLONG, M.A., Esq., Barrister-at-Law ; and J. W. MOORE, M.D., Diplomate in State Medicine and Ex-Scholar of Trin. Coll., Dublin ; Physician to the Meath Hospital ; Assistant Physician to Cork-street Fever Hospital.   Post 8vo., 336 pp.   7s. 6d.

This work embraces the following subjects :—

1. The Sanitary Duties imposed upon Officers and Authorities.— 2. A Summary and Index of Irish Sanitary Statutes.—3. Vital Statistics.—4. The Conditions necessary to Public Health.—5. Preventable Diseases.—6. Etiology of Disease.—7. Food ; Water Supply.—8. House Construction, Drainage, and Sewerage.—9. Hospital Accommodation.—10. Disinfection.—11. Meteorology.

The Principles of Surgery.

A Manual for Students ; specially useful to those preparing for Examinations in Surgery. BY JOHN A. ORR, F.R.C.S.I. ; formerly Surgeon to the City of Dublin Hospital.   Foolscap 8vo., 496 pp.   6s.

The Practice of Medical Electricity;

Showing the most Approved Apparatus, their methods of Use, and rules for the treatment of Nervous Diseases, more especially Paralysis and Neuralgia.   By G. D. POWELL, M.D., L.R.C.S.I., etc. Illustrated with Wood Engravings. Second edition, 8vo., cloth. 3s. 6d.

Lectures on the Clinical Uses of Electricity.

By WALTER G. SMITH, M.D. (Univ. Dub.); F.K. & Q.C.P. ; Assistant Physician to the Adelaide Hospital.   Foolscap 8vo., 54 pp., cloth.   1s. 6d.

Practical Remarks on the Treatment of Aneurism by Compression,

With plates of the Instruments hitherto employed in Dublin, and the recent improvements by Elastic Pressure. By JOLIFFE TUFFNELL, F.R.C.S. ; Fellow of the Royal Medical and Chirurgical Society of London ; Consulting Surgeon to the City of Dublin Hospital ; Surgeon to the Dublin District Military Prison, etc.   8vo., cloth.   6s.

By the same Author:

Practical Remarks on Stricture of the Rectum:

Its connection with Fistula in Ano, and Ulceration of the Bowel. 8vo. 1s.

By the same Author:

The Successful Treatment of the Internal Aneurism by Consolidation of the Contents of the Sac,

Illustrated by Cases in Hospital and Private Practice. Second edition, royal 8vo., with Coloured Plates. 5s.

Outlines of Zoology and Comparative Anatomy.

By MONTGOMERY A. WARD, M.B., M.Ch. (Univ. Dub.); Ex-Medical Scholar, T.C.D.; F.R.C.S.I.; Assistant Surgeon to the Adelaide Hospital; Demonstrator and Lecturer on Anatomy, Ledwich School of Medicine. Small 8vo., 150 pp., cloth. 8s. 6d.

This Manual has been specially compiled in a condensed form for those gentlemen who desire to prepare for the various examinations requiring the above subjects— *e.g.*, the Fellowships of the Royal College of Surgeons in England and Ireland; the M.D. of the Queen's University; and for Her Majesty's British, Indian, and Naval Medical Departments.

On Stricture of the Urethra,

Including an Account of the Perineal Abscess, Urinary Fistula, and Infiltration of the Urine. By SAMUEL G. WILMOT, M.D., F.R.C.S.; Consulting Surgeon to Steevens's Hospital; Consulting Surgeon to the Coombe Lying-in Hospital, etc. Post 8vo., cloth. 5s.

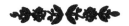

CPSIA information can be obtained
at www.ICGtesting.com
Printed in the USA
BVHW041155170119
538075BV00016B/395/P

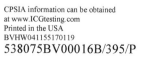

9 781332 837380